LSHTM

HLA and Disease

HLA and Disease

Edited by

Robert Lechler
Department of Immunology,
Royal Postgraduate Medical School,
London
UK

ACADEMIC PRESS
Harcourt Brace & Company, Publishers
London   Boston   San Diego   New York
Sydney   Tokyo

ACADEMIC PRESS LIMITED
24–28 Oval Road
LONDON NW1 7DX

U.S. Edition Published by
ACADEMIC PRESS INC.
San Diego, CA 92101

This book is printed on acid free paper

A catalogue record for this book is available from the British Library

ISBN 0–12–440320–4

Typeset by J&L Composition Ltd, Filey, North Yorkshire
Printed in Great Britain by The University Press, Cambridge

Contents

Contributors

Duncan Campbell
Department of Biochemistry
MRC Immunochemistry Unit
Oxford, England

Philip Dyer
Department of Medical Genetics
University of Manchester
Manchester, England

Robert Heard
Department of Neurology
Royal Prince Albert Hospital
New South Wales, Australia

Robert Lechler
Department of Immunology
Royal Postgraduate Medical School
London, England

Stephen Powis
Human Immunogenetics Laboratory
Imperial Cancer Research Fund
London, England

Alex So
Department of Rheumatology
Royal Postgraduate Medical School
London, England

John Trowsdale
Human Immunogenetics Laboratory
Imperial Cancer Research Fund
London, England

Mark Walport
Department of Rheumatology
Royal Postgraduate Medical School
London, England

Anthony Warrens
Department of Immunology
Royal Postgraduate Medical School
London, England

Foreword

J. Richard Batchelor

The initial driving force behind the investigation of the polymorphic HLA system was the expectation that matching an organ donor's HLA 'type' with that of the recipient would lead to improved allograft survival rates in clinical organ transplantation. Thus it came as a considerable surprise to most immunologists when major histocompatibility (MHC) molecules were discovered to be the structures to which the antigen-receptors of T lymphocytes bound, not merely in immune responses against incompatible tissues, but also in responses to other antigens. A comprehensive understanding of the structure and function of MHC molecules thereby became relevant not only to other branches of immunology, but also to clinical medicine and veterinary practice.

In the competitive world of scientific research, it is rather easy to forget group achievements, focusing, as we are prone to do, on the work of individual investigators. To my mind, the series of International Histocompatibility Workshops (IHWs) have been responsible for quite remarkable advances. In nearly 20 years between 1965 and 1984 the IHWs have been the vehicle by which the majority of HLA class I and class II polymorphisms were serologically identified, and their terminology agreed. With the introduction of recombinant DNA technology, the later IHWs have based HLA allele definition on nucleotide sequence. They have encouraged the development of the new technologies in many laboratories that, without the spur of having to produce reliable data for a Workshop deadline, might not have ventured into technologically unfamiliar territory. The result is that, although some gaps remain to be filled, sequence data for the majority of HLA polymorphisms are now available. All of us owe a considerable debt to the inspired leadership and hard work of the organizers of the IHWs.

What can we expect to gain from the acquisition of this information about the HLA system? Although MHC polymorphisms are not the only genetic factors governing immune responsiveness of a species, they are certainly amongst the strongest. We can therefore look forward to enlarging our understanding in two areas of great importance, namely, variation in immune protection to potentially persistent infective agents, and in autoimmune diseases. There is a real hope that the insights gained will result in clinical dividends. Already, recent work on immunity to *P. falciparum* malaria by Hill et al. (1992) has led to the recognition of a 9-mer peptide sequence from a liver-stage-specific antigen that binds to HLA-B53. This work not only provides a molecular basis for the protection afforded by HLA-B53 against severe *P. falciparum* malaria in the Gambia, but it also provides a vital clue to the producers of anti-malarial vaccines. It seems very likely that the same investigative strategy can be employed for other diseases caused by persistent infections.

Early studies on autoimmune diseases and HLA alleles were mainly designed to answer the question: does the autoimmune disease occur significantly more frequently in subjects with a particular HLA phenotype? To take matters further requires further questions to be asked, and will entail longer term research commitment. For example, in many autoimmune states it is necessary to distinguish between an MHC-linked susceptibility to *acquisition* of the initial disease and an MHC-linked susceptibility to *progression* of the disease process. Rheumatoid arthritis is an interesting example of this problem. Virtually all the earliest studies involved HLA typing of classical cases, defined by criteria of the American Rheumatism Association. Striking associations were described with HLA-DR4 and DR1. However, the Norfolk Arthritis Registry, a community-based incidence study of early rheumatoid arthritis, has already found that there is no increase in the frequencies of DR4 and DR1 in patients with early arthritis (Thomson et al., 1993). The inference is that the disease-associated alleles exert their effect on progression of early arthritis to classical rheumatoid arthritis. Following such clues will require long-term studies and agencies supporting such research need to be aware of this.

It is therefore timely that a book should be written bringing together not only the genetics and structural information on HLA but also an explanation of these data in terms of function. The insights this gives us into immune responsiveness and the pathogenesis of autoimmune diseases are exciting.

I congratulate the editor and authors of this volume for providing an excellent and up-to-date summary of current knowledge on the HLA system and its role in the pathogenesis of important diseases.

References

Hill, A.V.S., Elvin, J., Willis, A.C. et al. (1992). Molecular analysis of the association of HLA-B53 and resistance to severe malaria. *Nature* **360**: 434–439.

Thomson, W., Pepper, L., Payton, A. et al. (1993). Absence of an association between HLA-DRB1*04 and rheumatoid arthritis in newly diagnosed cases from the community. *Ann. Rheum. Dis.* (in press).

Introduction

Robert Lechler

The major histocompatibility complex (MHC), referred to in man as the HLA (human leucocyte antigen) region, has been one of the most intensively studied genetic regions during the past two decades. As a consequence of the application of modern cloning techniques, the HLA region is on the brink of full characterization and, together with recent advances in immunology, this creates the possibility of making significant progress in understanding the mechanisms responsible for the well-known associations of certain HLA types with human disease.

The MHC has been explored in several species, most notably in man and mouse, and is highly conserved. One of the conclusions that has emerged from recent cloning efforts is that the MHC is probably the area of the mammalian genome that is most densely populated with functional genes. Current estimates are that the region contains in the order of 200 genes. These include, of course, the genes encoding the MHC class I and class II molecules. The MHC genes are the most polymorphic of all mammalian genes. The functional significance of this sequence variation, and its possible relationship to disease susceptibility is one of the topics discussed in this book. In addition there are a large number of other genes, some with known functions and some whose functions are as yet unidentified. Some of the well-characterized genes encode proteins with obvious relevance to the immune system. These include three complement genes, the tumour necrosis factor genes, and a cluster of genes that appear to be involved in the digestion of antigens inside antigen-presenting cells and the loading of antigen fragments on to MHC molecules for subsequent antigen presentation. Less is known of the polymorphism of these recently discovered genes but it may prove to be the case that sequence variation at one or more of these loci predisposes to autoimmune disease.

The first reports of an association between an HLA antigen and disease were those of Hodgkin's lymphoma with a cross-reactive group of HLA-B antigens, B5, B15, B18 and B35 (Amiel, 1967) and of acute lymphoblastic leukaemia with HLA-A2 (Walford et al., 1970). These particular associations have not proven to be consistently reproducible, but a short time later the remarkable association between the rheumatological disorder, ankylosing spondylitis, and HLA-B27 was described

(Brewerton et al., 1973; Schlosstein et al., 1973). These observations provided the impetus for further studies of HLA and disease associations, and a large number of diseases have been shown to be associated with the possession of particular HLA types. The aim of this book is to provide a framework within which to interpret HLA and disease associations, and to design further studies.

The book is divided into two sections, A and B. Section A presents the current state of knowledge of the genetics and the structure of the HLA antigens. These topics are covered in Chapters 1 and 2. In Chapters 3 and 4 the biology of MHC molecules is discussed, with particular emphasis on the ways in which MHC antigens contribute to immune recognition and immune regulation. Section B begins with a consideration of the mechanisms underlying HLA and disease associations, in the light of the earlier discussions of the structure and functions of the MHC molecules (Chapter 5). Chapter 6 describes the principles of designing and interpreting an HLA and disease study, followed in Chapter 7 by a detailed description of some of the best characterized associations of HLA antigens with diseases that are thought to have an autoimmune pathogenesis. Chapter 8 focuses on a series of connective tissue diseases, some of which are more closely linked with the HLA class III region, an area that includes the genes for the complement proteins, C2, C4 and Factor B. Finally, in Chapter 9, the very exciting discoveries of the many additional genes within the MHC, some with important immune functions, are presented. Their possible relevance to disease pathogenesis is discussed.

The value of defining HLA and disease associations can be thought of in two ways. The first is that the definition of an association may help to define an 'at risk' population. This can be translated into practical benefit if a means of prevention becomes available. The second benefit of defining genetic susceptibility factors in any disease is that this can shed light on the mechanisms underlying the disease. This, in turn, can pave the way for more precisely targeted strategies for disease prevention or treatment.

There has never been a more exciting time for studies of this kind. The advent of new techniques for the precise definition of HLA polymorphisms, and the detailed molecular definition of how MHC molecules present antigens to T lymphocytes, and of how sequence variation influences this process, provides a conceptual context within which HLA and disease associations can be understood. As the autoantigens that are aberrantly recognized in autoimmune disease states are characterized, existing hypotheses can be tested directly. Furthermore, the discovery of the many additional genes within the HLA region creates new possibilities for identifying genetic susceptibility factors.

References

Amiel, J.L. (1967). *Histocompatibility Testing 1967* (eds E.S. Curtoni, P.L. Mattiuz and R.M. Tosi), pp. 79–81, Munksgaard, Copenhagen.

Brewerton, D.A., Caffrey, M., Hart, F.D. et al. (1973). Ankylosing spondylitis and HL-A27. *Lancet* **1**: 904–907.

Schlosstein, L., Terasaki, P.I., Bluestone, J. et al. (1973). High association of a HL-A antigen, w27, with ankylosing spondylitis. *N. Engl. J. Med.* **288**: 704–706.

Walford, R.L., Finkelstein, S., Neerhout, R. et al. (1970). Acute childhood leukemia in relation to the HL-A human transplantation genes. *Nature* **225**: 461-462.

CHAPTER 1

Genetics, polymorphism and regulation of expression of HLA region genes

Alex So

Department of Rheumatology
Royal Postgraduate Medical School
London, UK

Introduction

The HLA (human leucocyte antigen) molecules are encoded by genes located within the major histocompatibility complex (MHC). Cytogenetic studies have mapped the MHC region to the p21.3 band on the short arm of chromosome 6, where it spans some four million base pairs of DNA. This complex region contains multiple expressed and non-expressed genes arranged in three major gene clusters. The class I region contains genes which encode the classical transplantation antigens HLA-A, B and C. The class II region contains genes encoding the HLA-D molecules (HLA-DR, DQ and DP). The class III region contains the genes encoding complement proteins Factor B, C2 and C4, and the cytochrome P-450 enzyme steroid 21-hydroxylase. Additional genes which have recently been localized to this region include tumour necrosis factor (TNF α and β), the 70 kD heat shock proteins (HSP70), peptide transporters and proteasome genes. The region is remarkable in the high degree of genetic polymorphism at many of the loci. Polymorphism is defined as a Mendelian trait that is present in the population in at least two phenotypes, each occurring with a frequency of greater than 1%. The HLA antigens form the most polymorphic antigen system in man. The discovery of the HLA system dates back to the early 1950s, based on the studies of Dausset, Payne, van Rood, and others who described the presence of leucocyte-agglutinating antisera in polytransfused individuals and multiparous women (Dausset, 1954; Payne, 1958; van Rood, 1962). These antigens were shown subsequently to be extremely polymorphic, and were encoded by a series of closely linked genetic loci mapped to chromosome 6,

HLA and Disease
ISBN 0–12–440320–4

which we now recognize as the class I genes. These discoveries were paralleled by the identification of H-2, the murine homologue of the HLA system. It was identified by the pioneering experiments of Gorer and Snell, who demonstrated that tumour graft rejection between inbred strains of mice was under genetic control and that rejection was associated with the development of antibodies against alloantigens present on leucocytes. In humans, a correlation between graft rejection and HLA compatibility was also observed in organ transplantation; hence the genetic region encoding these alloantigens was named the major histocompatibility complex. Later investigators demonstrated that genes within the MHC also controlled the allogeneic mixed lymphocyte response (MLR) (Bach and Hirschhorn, 1964), which we now know to result from differences in the class II antigens. As transplantation is obviously not a normal physiological event, a clue to the function of these histocompatibility molecules came from the work of McDevitt and his colleagues, who mapped the genes responsible for genetically determined variation in immune reactivity to the MHC region in mice (McDevitt et al., 1972). We now know that the primary biological role of HLA molecules is in the regulation of immune responses to foreign antigens, and the discrimination of self from non-self.

Some of the major historical landmarks in the discovery of the MHC and of its functions are summarized in Table 1.1.

Physical map of the MHC

The human MHC spans 3800 kb of DNA. The orientation of the three major gene clusters on chromosome 6, and their relationship with one another was first clarified by genomic cloning and subsequently by pulse-field gel electrophoresis, a technique

Table 1.1   Historical landmarks in the discovery of the HLA system

Year	Investigators	Discovery
1936	Gorer (1936)	Genetic basis of tumour rejection in mice and identification of antisera specific for MHC antigens
1958	Snell (1958)	Generation of MHC congenic strains of mice that enabled dissection of the genetics of the H-2 system
1954–1962	Dausset (1954), Payne and Rolfs (1958), van Rood (1962)	Identification of HLA antigens using alloantisera and establishment of the International HLA Workshops
1964	Bach and Hirschhorn (1964)	Mixed lymphocyte reaction
1972	McDevitt et al. (1972)	Mapping of immune response (*Ir*) genes to the MHC in mice
1974	Zinkernagel and Doherty (1974)	MHC restriction of cytotoxic T-cells
1976	Terhorst et al. (1976)	Partial protein sequence of HLA-A2
1980	Ploegh et al. (1980)	cDNA cloning and sequencing of class I gene
1982	Lee et al. (1982)	cDNA cloning of DRα chain
1987	Bjorkman et al. (1987)	X-Ray crystal structure of HLA-A2

which allows separation of large DNA fragments for construction of restriction maps (Hardy et al., 1986; Dunham et al., 1987; Lawrance et al., 1987; Spies et al., 1989; Sargent et al., 1989). Combining the results obtained using these techniques, a physical map of the MHC has been produced, with the HLA-DP locus at the centromeric end, and the HLA-A locus at the telomeric end. The region contains a very large number of transcribed genes; the functions of some of these genes has yet to be defined. The genetic organization of the HLA complex is shown in Figure 1.1, first in a simplified form to illustrate the physical relationship between the class I, II, and III regions, followed by a comprehensive map that includes the many newly identified genes that reside within the MHC complex. The physical structure of the genes encoding HLA class I and II genes will be discussed in further detail.

Identification of polymorphism

One of the hallmarks of the HLA gene products is the high degree of polymorphism they exhibit. There are multiple alleles at each locus and each genetic region contains several related genes at different loci. As more sophisticated methods of studying molecular structure have developed, so the complexity of the polymorphic variations have become apparent. Serological reagents remain an important tool for the detection of polymorphism and, in addition to polyclonal antisera, which continue to be the mainstay of HLA-typing, monoclonal reagents against HLA class I and class II antigens are now widely available. Based on the phenomenon of the mixed lymphocyte reaction, in which lymphocytes from individuals who differ in their HLA-D region proliferate when cultured in vitro, cellular typing has been used to define alleles within serologically identical groups of class II (HLA-D) alleles. To distinguish between the specificities defined by these two methods, HLA-D region allelic variations detected by serology and cellular techniques are identified by the prefixes DR and Dw, respectively.

In the last ten years, biochemical and molecular biological techniques have provided further detailed information on the fine structure of HLA molecules and the genes which encode them. Isoelectric focusing, two-dimensional gel electrophoresis, and amino-acid sequencing detect charge and sequence differences between class I and class II alleles. With the cloning of HLA genes from genomic and cDNA libraries, the primary structure of the molecules and their genetic organization can be deduced from their DNA sequence. The availability of probes for the individual genes of interest has allowed restriction fragment length polymorphism (RFLP) analysis, which has detected considerable variation in the patterns of hybridizing fragments in most of the genes studied. This system of analysis has been studied in greatest detail for the HLA-D region genes; the class I genes have been more difficult to analyse, because of the complexity of the RFLPs generated.

More recently, the polymerase chain reaction (PCR) technique of amplifying DNA sequences has provided a rapid method for the cloning and sequencing of genes and has enabled a detailed analysis of molecular polymorphism of a large number of HLA alleles. From the DNA sequences, allele-specific oligonucleotide probes have been synthesized and used to identify HLA genotypes in hybridization experiments.

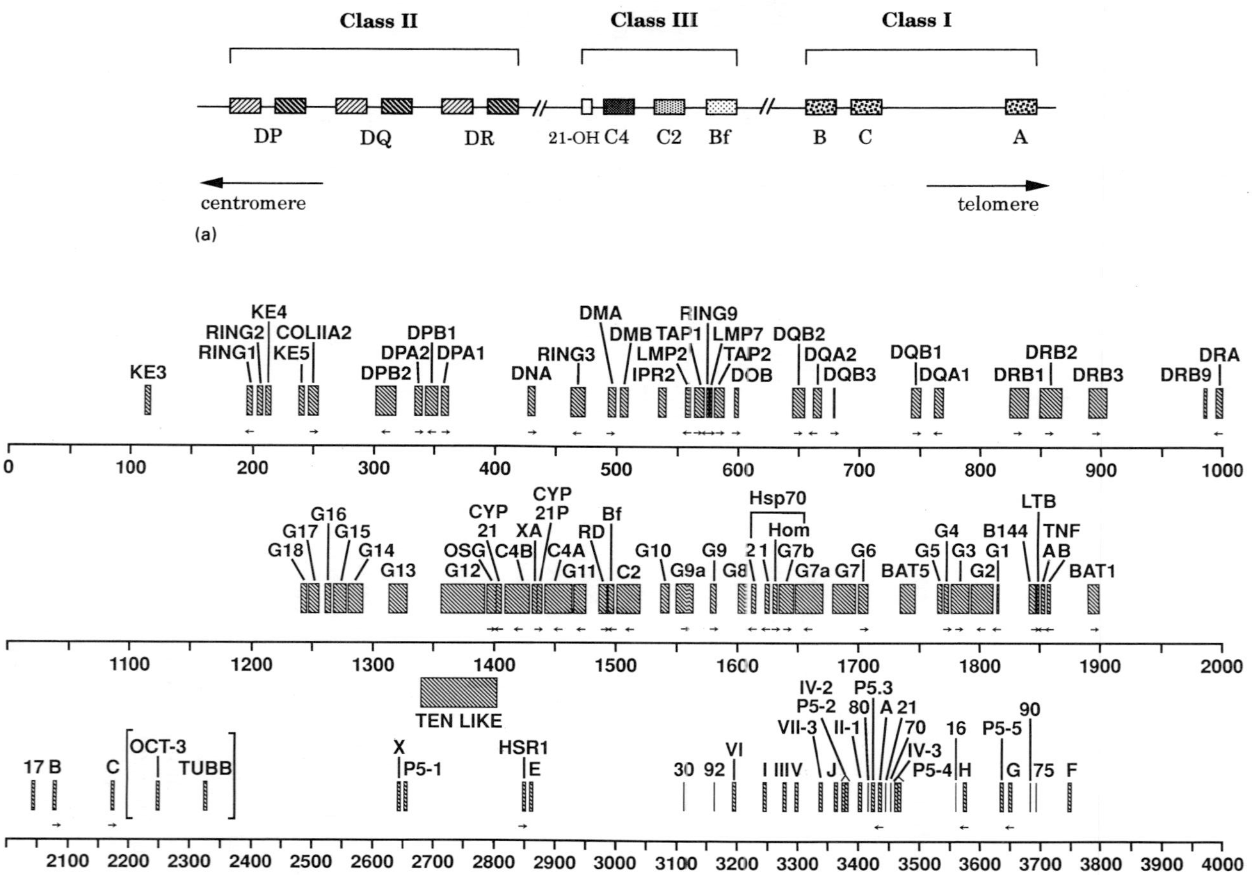

Figure 1.1 (a) The arrangement of the three major regions of the HLA region are shown; the distances between the loci are not to scale. (b) Map of the human major histocompatibility complex.

Table 1.2   Designations of HLA-A, -B and -C alleles.

HLA alleles[a]	HLA specificity	HLA alleles[a]	HLA specificity
A*0101	A1	B*1801	B18
A*0201	A2	B*2701	B27
A*0202	A2	B*2702	B27
A*0203	A203	B*2703	B27
A*0204	A2	B*2704	B27
A*0205	A2	B*2705	B27
A*0206	A2	B*2706	B27
A*0207	A2	**B*2707**	B27
A*0208	A2	B*3501	B35
A*0209	A2	B*3502	B35
A*0210	A210	**B*3503**	B35
A*0211	A2	**B*3504**	B35
A*0212	A2	**B*3505**	B35
A*0301	A3	**B*3506**	B35
A*0302	A3	B*3701	B37
A*1101	A11	B*3801	B38(16)
A*1102	A11	B*3901	B3901
A*2301	A23(9)	**B*3902**	B3902
A*2401	A24(9)	B*4001	B60(40)
A*2402	A24(9)	B*4002	B40
A*2403	A2403	**B*4003**	B40
A*2501	A25(10)	**B*4004**	B40
A*2601	A26(10)	**B*4005**	B4005
A*2901	A29(19)	B*4101	B41
A*2902	A29(19)	B*4201	B42
A*3001	A30(19)	B*4401	B44(12)
A*3002	A30(19)	B*4402	B44(12)
A*31011[b]	A31(19)	**B*4403**	B44(12)
A*31012	A31(19)	**B*4501**	B45(12)
A*3201	A32(19)	B*4601	B46
A*3301	A33(19)	B*4701	B47
A*3401	A34(10)	**B*4801**	B48
A*3402	A34(10)	B*4901	B49(21)
A*3601	A36	**B*5001**	B50(21)
A*4301	A43	B*5101	B51(5)
A*6601	A66(10)	**B*5102**	B5102
A*6602	A66(10)	**B*5103**	B5103
A*6801	A68(28)	B*5201	B52(5)
A*6802	A68(28)	B*5301	B53
A*6901	A69(28)	**B*5401**	B54(22)
A*7401	A74(19)	**B*5501**	B55(22)
B.0701	B7	**B*5502**	B55(22)
B*0702	B7	**B*5601**	B56(22)
B*0703	B703	**B*5602**	B56(22)
B*0801	B8	B*5701	B57(17)
B*1301	B13	**B*5702**	B57(17)
B*1302	B13	B*5801	B58(17)
B*1401	B14	B*7801	B7801
B*1402	B65(14)	**B*7901**	—
B*1501	B62(15)	Cw*0101	Cw1
B*1502	B75(15)	**Cw*0102**	Cw1
B*1503	B72(70)	Cw*0201	Cw2
B*1504	B62(15)	Cw*02021	Cw2

Table 1.2   Continued

HLA alleles[a]	HLA specificity	HLA alleles[a]	HLA specificity
Cw*02022	Cw2	**DRB1*1306**	DR13(6)
Cw*0301	Cw3	DRB1*1401	DR14(6)
Cw*0302	Cw3	DRB1*1402	DR14(6)
Cw*0401	Cw4	DRB1*1403	DR1403
Cw*0501	Cw5	DRB1*1404	DR1404
Cw*0601	Cw6	DRB1*1405	DR14(6)
Cw*0701	Cw7	**DRB1*1406**	DR14(6)
Cw*0702	Cw7	**DRB1*1407**	DR14(6)
Cw*0801	Cw8	**DRB1*1408**	DR14(6)
Cw*0802	Cw8	**DRB1*1409**	DR14(6)
Cw*1201	—	**DRB1*1410**	—
Cw*1202	—	DRB1*0701	DR7
Cw*1301	—	DRB1*0702	DR7
Cw*1401	—	DRB1*0801	DR8
DRA*0101	—	DRB1*08021	DR8
DRA*0102	—	DRB1*08022	DR8
DRB1*0101	DR1	DRB1*08031	DR8
DRB1*0102	DR1	DRB1*08032	DR8
DRB1*0103	DR103	DRB1*0804	DR8
DRB1*1501	DR15(2)	**DRB1*0805**	DR8
DRB1*1502	DR15(2)	DRB1*09011	DR9
DRB1*1503	DR15(2)	DRB1*09012	DR9
DRB1*1601	DR16(2)	DRB1*1001	DR10
DRB1*1602	DR16(2)	DRB3*0101	DR52
DRB1*0301	DR17(3)	DRB3*0201	DR52
DRB1*0302	DR18(3)	DRB3*0202	DR52
DRB1*0303	DR18(3)	DRB3*0301	DR52
DRB1*0401	DR4	DRB4*0101	DR53
DRB1*0402	DR4	DRB5*0101	DR51
DRB1*0403	DR4	DRB5*0102	DR51
DRB1*0404	DR4	DRB5*0201	DR51
DRB1*0405	DR4	DRB5*0202	DR51
DRB1*0406	DR4	**DRB6*0101**	—
DRB1*0407	DR4	**DRB6*0201**	—
DRB1*0408	DR4	**DRB6*0202**	—
DRB1*0409	DR4	DQA1*0101	—
DRB1*0410	DR4	DQA1*0102	—
DRB1*0411	DR4	DQA1*0103	—
DRB1*0412	DR4	**DQA1*0104**	—
DRB1*11011	DR11(5)	DQA1*0201	—
DRB1*11012	DR11(5)	DQA1*03011	—
DRB1*1102	DR11(5)	DQA1*03012	—
DRB1*1103	DR11(5)	DQA1*0302	—
DRB1*11041	DR11(5)	DQA1*0401	—
DRB1*11042	DR11(5)	DQA1*0501[c]	—
DRB1*1105	DR11(5)	DQA1*05011	—
DRB1*1201	DR12(5)	DQA1*05012	—
DRB1*1202	DR12(5)	DQA1*05013	—
DRB1*1301	DR13(6)	DQA1*0601	—
DRB1*1302	DR13(6)	DQB1*0501	DQ5(1)
DRB1*1303	DR13(6)	DQB1*0502	DQ5(1)
DRB1*1304	DR13(6)	DQB1*05031	DQ5(1)
DRB1*1305	DR13(6)	DQB1*05032	DQ5(1)

Table 1.2 Continued

HLA alleles[a]	HLA specificity	HLA alleles[a]	HLA specificity
DQB1*0504	—	DPB1*0501	DPw5
DQB1*0601	DQ6(1)	DPB1*0601	DPw6
DQB1*0602	DQ6(1)	DPB1*0801	—
DQB1*0603	DQ6(1)	DPB1*0901	—
DQB1*0604	DQ6(1)	DPB1*1001	—
DQB1*0605	DQ6(1)	DPB1*1101	—
DQB1*0606	—	DPB1*1301	—
DQB1*0201	DQ2	DPB1*1401	—
DQB1*0301	DQ7(3)	DPB1*1501	—
DQB1*0302	DQ8(3)	DPB1*1601	—
DQB1*03031	DQ9(3)	DPB1*1701	—
DQB1*03032	DQ9(3)	DPB1*1801	—
DQB1*0304	DQ7(3)	DPB1*1901	—
DQB1*0401	DQ4	**DPB1*2001**	—
DQB1*0402	DQ4	**DPB1*2101**	—
DPA1*0101	—	**DPB1*2201**	—
DPA1*0102	—	**DPB1*2301**	—
DPA1*0103	—	**DPB1*2401**	—
DPA1*0201	—	**DPB1*2501**	—
DPA1*02021	—	**DPB1*2601**	—
DPA1*02022	—	**DPB1*2701**	—
DPA1*0301	—	**DPB1*2801**	—
DPA1*0401	—	**DPB1*2901**	—
DPB1*0101	DPw1	**DPB1*3001**	—
DPB1*0201	DPw2	**DPB1*3101**	—
DPB1*02011	DPw2	**DPB1*3201**	—
DPB1*02012	DPw2	**DBP1*3301**	—
DPB1*0202	DPw2	**DPB1*3401**	—
DPB1*0301	DPw3	**DPB1*3501**	—
DPB1*0401	DPw4	**DBP1*3601**	—
DPB1*0402	DPw4		

[a] Allele names given in bold type are newly assigned.
[b] This sequence has been previously assigned with a four-digit allele name.
[c] This sequence can only be assigned a four-digit allele name, as it is either published only as a protein or partial nucleotide sequence.

Over the last 20 years, the co-ordination of an international collaborative effort to study the HLA system has been undertaken through a series of International Histocompatibility Workshops. The techniques that are in current use for the definition of HLA polymorphism are discussed in more detail in Chapter 6.

Nomenclature

With the recognition of the increasing number of genes and alleles which are present within the MHC, the nomenclature of the genes and their products are constantly under revision. In accordance with internationally accepted genetic nomenclature, the locus is indicated first, followed by the identification number of the allele, separated from the designation of the locus by an asterisk. Therefore, HLA-A2 is designated as HLA-A*02, and the ten known subtypes of A2 are identified as A*0201 to A*0210. The different HLA class I genes are denoted by a suffix: HLA-A to HLA-G: HLA class II genes are indicated by the subregion of localization (DR, DQ, DO, DN or DP), and whether they encode the α chain sequences (e.g. HLA DRA) or β chain sequences (e.g. HLA DRB). The same system of allele identification as outlined above for class I genes is used. At recent meetings of the nomenclature committee in 1989 and 1991 a revised list was produced which took into account new alleles defined by nucleotide and inferred amino-acid sequences (Bodmer et al., 1990, 1992), which is displayed in Table 1.2.

HLA class I genes

Structure of class I antigens

HLA class I antigens are heterodimeric membrane-bound glycoproteins made up of a heavy chain of 45 kD, which is non-covalently associated with beta-2-microglobulin (β2m). β2m is a 12 kD serum protein which is encoded by a gene on chromosome 15. A schematic diagram of the structure of MHC class I and class II molecules is shown in Figure 1.2. The two chains of the class I molecule associate in the endoplasmic reticulum and are then transported to the cell surface. The heavy chain consists of 340 amino acids and has three membrane-external domains (α1, α2, and α3), each of which consist of approximately 90 amino acids. The transmembrane region consists of 25–30 hydrophobic amino acids, and the intracytoplasmic portion consists of a further 25–30 amino acids. The α2 and α3 domains have intrachain disulphide bonds between cysteine residues at 101 and 164, and 203 and 259, respectively, and a glycosylation site is found at position 86 within the α1 domain. There is extensive allelic polymorphism of HLA-A, -B, and -C genes, with the majority of the polymorphic differences present in the α1 and α2 domains (for more details, see Chapter 2). The α3 domain shows sequence homology to immunoglobulin CH3 constant region domains (Travers et al., 1984), indicating that HLA genes have evolved from ancestral immunoglobulin-like genes.

Recently, the three-dimensional structure of a number of HLA alleles including HLA-A*0201, HLA-A*6801 and HLA-B*2705 have been solved by X-ray crystallography (discussed further in Chapter 2). The molecule has an antigen-binding cleft which is approximately 25Å by 10Å. It is formed by a floor of eight anti-parallel β-pleated sheets, flanked by side walls of α-helices. Both α1 and α2 domains contribute to the formation of the antigen-binding site, and are supported by the α3 domain and β2m (Figure 1.2).

Genetic organization

There are multiple class I genes in the MHC (Figure 1.1). Those which encode the HLA-A, B and C antigens have also been termed classical class I genes, and the

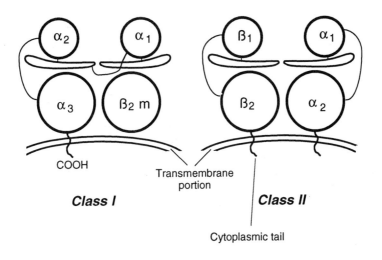

Figure 1.2 Schematic diagram of MHC class I and class II molecules. The overall structural similarity of the two classes of molecule is illustrated. In both cases the two membrane-proximal domains have the features of immunoglobulin domains, and the membrane-distal domains are organized into a platform of anti-parallel strands on which lies a stretch of α-helical sequence. The major differences between the two classes of MHC molecule are that the domains are distributed asymmetrically in class I molecules, such that the heavy chain has three domains, co-expressed with the single domain of β2 microglobulin. In contrast, the two chains of the class II molecule both have two domains. An additional difference is that both chains of the class II molecule are inserted into the cell membrane, whereas only the heavy chain of the class I molecule spans the cell membrane.

others non-classical. The products of the classical class I genes are so called because they play a central role in T-cell recognition by binding and displaying peptides for recognition by CD8$^+$ T-cells (discussed below). Seventeen class I and class I-like genes have been identified within the MHC, and six of them are associated with transcribed products. The remaining 11 are pseudogenes, as they have various deleterious mutations in the DNA sequence which prevent transcription, or are only fragments of an entire gene. Genetic mapping based on recombination fractions places HLA-B 0.2 cM centromeric to HLA-C, and HLA-A 0.8 cM telomeric to HLA-C, and this organization is in good agreement with the physical mapping results (Koller et al., 1989) (1 cM has been calculated to span 1×10^6 bp of DNA). From pulse-field gel electrophoresis studies, the class I region of the MHC spans approximately 1.4×10^6 base pairs, and lies 0.65×10^6 base pairs telomeric to the C2 gene, which lies at the telomeric end of the class III region.

HLA class I genes share a very similar organization. They consist of eight exons, and the exon–intron organization reflects the domain structure of the molecule (Figure 1.3). The first exon encodes the signal sequence, and the second, third, and fourth exons the α1, α2, and α3 domains, respectively. The transmembrane region is

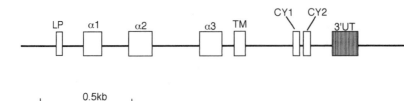

Figure 1.3   Genomic organization of the HLA class I gene Bw58 (Ways et al., 1985). Exons are indicated in open boxes. LP=leader peptide; TM=transmembrane domain; CY=cytoplasmic domain; 3'UT=3'-untranslated sequence.

encoded by the fifth exon, and the cytoplasmic tail (including the 3-untranslated region) by exons 6–8. Fine differences are observed between the different class I loci: HLA-B locus molecules have no coding sequences on exon 8, and HLA-A and -B genes possess three more nucleotides in exon 5 compared to HLA-C.

In addition to the classical class I genes, non-classical genes within the MHC include HLA-E, -F, and -G, and an as yet unclassified gene known as HA2 (Orr, 1989). These genes are the human homologues of the murine Qa/TL genes, which have a restricted range of tissue expression. HLA-E is located between HLA-B and -C, and HLA-F and -G telomeric to HLA-A, separated from HLA-A by a recombination distance of 8.0 cM (Koller et al., 1989). By sequence, there is strong homology between these molecules and the classical class I antigens (over 80% at the protein level), but it is unclear whether they exhibit any significant polymorphism. The patterns of expression of the major classical and non-classical class I antigens are summarized in Table 1.3.

Table 1.3   HLA class I antigens and their expression

Antigen	Distribution
Classical	
HLA-A	
HLA-B	Present on most nucleated cells; low expression by myocardium, and skeletal muscle. Not detected on CNS neurones and villous trophoblast
HLA-C	
Non-classical	
HLA-E	Resting peripheral T-cells
HLA-F	Not known
HLA-G	Chorionic cytotrophoblast

Polymorphism of class I genes

The HLA class I molecules show extensive polymorphism at each of the classical loci. At the Nomenclature meeting following the 11th International Workshop, 41 distinct HLA-A, 61 HLA-B, and 18 HLA-C alleles were recognized (Bodmer et al., 1992). The frequency of individual alleles in a population varies according to the ethnic group and the population studied, for example, HLA-A2 is found in 45% of the European Caucasoid population, but in African blacks, the frequency is only 20%. Conversely, HLA-Bw52 is present in 20.5% of the Japanese population but the

```
α1 domain     ▼                           ▼       ▼ ▼▼▼ ▼▼▼ ▼ ▼▼ ▼
              1        10        20        30        40        50        60        70        80        90
consensus GSHSMRYFYTSVSRPGRGEPRFIAVGYVDDTQFVRFDSDAASPRMEPRAPWIEQEGPEYWDRETQIVKAQSQTDRESLRTLRGYYNQSEA
    A2.1  --------F------------------------------Q-----------------G--RK---H---H-VD-G----------
    A2.2Y -------------------------------------R-----------------G--RK---H---H-VD-G----------
    A2.2F --------F----------------------------R-----------------G--RK---H---H-VD-G----------
    A2.3  --------F------------------------------Q-----------------G--RK---H---H-VD-G----------
    A2.4a ---------------------------------------Q-----------------G--RK---H---H-VD-G----------
    A2.4b --------F------------------------------Q-----------------G--RK---H---H-VD-G----------
    Aw69  ---------------------------------------Q-----------------N-RN--------VD-G----------
    Aw68.2 -----------H---------------------------Q-----------------N-RN--------VD-G----------
    Aw68.1 --------------------------------------Q-----------------N-RN--------VD-G----------
    A3.1  --------F------------------------------Q-----------------Q--RN--------VD-G----------
    A3.2  --------F------------------------------Q-----------------Q--RN--------VD-G----------
    A11   ---------------------------------------Q-----------------Q--RN--------VD-G---------D
    A1    --------F----------------------------QK------------------Q--RNM--H-----AN-G--------D
    A32   --------F------------------------------Q-----------------Q--RN---H---------IALR-------
    Aw24  --------S------------------------------Q-----------------E--GK---H------N--IALR-------
    Bw58  ----------AM-----------------------T---------------------G--RNM--SA--Y--N--IALR-------
    B27.1 --------H------------T------L---------E-------------------C--KA----D----LR-------
    B27.2 --------H------------T------L---------E-------------------C--KA-----N--IALR-------
    B27.3 --------H------------T------L---------E-------------------C--KA---------LR-------
    B27.4 --------H------------T------L---------E-------------------C--KA---------LR-------
    B27f  --------H------------T------L---------E-------------------C--KA--Y--N---ALR-------
    B44.1 ----------AM---------T------L------T---K-----------------S-TNT--Y--N---AAR-------
    B44.2 ----------AM---------T------L------T---K-----------------S-TNT--Y--N---ALR-------
    B13   ----------AM---------T-------------T----A----------------S-TNT--Y--N---ALR-------
    Bw47  ----------AM---------T------L------T---K-----------------S-TNT--Y--N---LR-------
    Bw65  ----------A----------S-------------E---------------------N--C-TNT-------N---------
    B14   ---------------------S-------------E---------------------N--C-TNT-------N---------
    B18   --------H------------S----G--------T---------------------N---S-TNT--Y-----N---------
    B40*  --------H------------T------L------T---K-----------------S-TNT--Y-----N---------
    Bw41  --------H-AM---------T------L------T---K-----------------S-TNT--Y-----N---------
    Bw60  --------H-AM---------T------L------T---K-----------------S-TNT--Y-----N---------
    B8    --------D-AM---------S-------------E---------------------N---F-TNT-------N---------
    Bw42  ---------------------S-------------E---------------------N--Y---A-------N---------
    B7.1  ---------------------S-------------E---------------------N--Y---A-------N---------
    B7.2  ---------------------S-------------E---------------------N--Y---A-------N---------
    Cw1   C----K--F------------S------------G------V------------KY-R-A----V---N---------
    Cw2.1 C--------A---S----H--------------G---GR-V------------KY-R-A----VN--K---------
    Cw2.2 C----------A---S----H-------------G------V------------KY-R-A----VN--K---------
    Cw3   -------C-A---------H--------------DE---G------V-RK----------KY-P-A----V---N---------
consensus GSHSMRYFYTSVSRPGRGEPRFIAVGYVDDTQFVRFDSDAASPRMEPRAPWIEQEGPEYWDRETQIVKAQSQTDRESLRTLRGYYNQSEA
              1        10        20        30        40        50        60        70        80        90
```

Figure 1.4 (a) Amino-acid sequences of 15 HLA-A, 20 -B, and four -C molecules in the α1, α2, and α3 domains (Parham et al., 1989a). Each sequence is compared with a consensus sequence constructed from the most frequent amino acid at each position. Dashes indicate identity with the consensus. Continued on pages 12 and 13.

frequency is 3% in Caucasoids (Baur and Danilovs, 1980b). Even within one ethnic group, the frequency of a particular allele may vary depending on the geographic location, for example, HLA-B8 is found in 30% of the UK Caucasoid population while in southern Europe its frequency is 14% (Tiwari and Terasaki, 1985).

The structural basis of allelic polymorphism has been addressed directly by comparison of protein and nucleotide sequences of more than 100 recognized alleles of HLA-A, -B, and -C loci. A representative sample of amino-acid sequences of HLA class I molecules is presented in Figure 1.4, together with a Kabat–Wu plot to illustrate the clustering of polymorphic positions in these molecules. From these analyses, it is clear that polymorphism is predominantly due to amino-acid changes in the α1 and α2 domains of the molecule. The α3 and transmembrane regions are also polymorphic but much less so. When the positions of allelic amino-acid substitutions in the α1 and α2 domains are superimposed upon the crystallographic structure of HLA-A2, it is evident that most of the substitutions are clustered around the antigen-binding cleft and are located either in the floor or the side walls of the

```
α2 domain      ▼ ▼              ▼ ▼                                              ▼       ▼
             100        110        120        130        140        150        160        170        180
consensus GSHTLQRMYGCDVGPDGRLLRGYHQYAYDGKDYIALNEDLRSWTAADTAAQITQRKWEAARVAEQLRAYLEGTCVEWLRRYLENGKETLQRA
    A2.1  ----V--------S-W-F----------------K---------M---T-KH----H------------------------------T
    A2.2Y -------------S-W-F----------------K---------M---T-KH----H----W-------------------------T
    A2.2F -------------S-W-F----------------K---------M---T-KH----H----W-------------------------T
    A2.3  ----V--------S-W-F----------------K---------M---T-KH---T-HE---W-------------------------T
    A2.4a ----V--------S-W-F----------------K---------M---T-KH----H------------------------------T
    A2.4b ----V---C----S-W-F----------------K---------M---T-KH----H------------------------------T
    Aw69  ----V--------S-W-F----------------K---------M---T-KH----H------------------------------T
    Aw68.2 ----I-----------F-----------------K---------M---T-KH----H----W-------------------------T
    Aw68.1 ----I-M-------S----F----R-D-------K---------M---T-KH----H----W-------------------------T
    A3.1  ----I-I-------S---F----R-D------------------M-----K-----HE--------D--------------------T
    A3.2  ----I-I-------S---F----R-D------------------M-----K-----H----Q----D--------------------T
    A11   ----I-I---------F----R-D--------------------M-----K-----HA---Q--------R----------------T
    A1    ----I-I---------F----R-D--------------------M-----K-----VHA--R-V----R--DG--------------T
    A32   ----I-M-------------Q-D---------------------M-----------------------------------------
    Aw24  ------M-F-----S---F----------------K---------M-----K-----H----Q--------DG--------------
    Bw58  ---II-------L---------HD-S----------------S-------------------------L-------------------
    B27.1 ------N--------------D--------------------S------------------E--------------------------
    B27.2 ------N--------------D--------------------S------------------E--------------------------
    B27.3 ------N--------------D--------------------S----------E-------E--------------------------
    B27.4 ------N----------------D------------------S----------E-------E--------------------------
    B27f  ------N--------------D--------------------S------------------E--------------------------
    B44.1 ---II----------------D-D------------------S-----------------D-----L---S-----------------
    B44.2 ---II----------------D-D------------------S-----------------D-----L---S-----------------
    B13   ----W-T----L---------HN-L----------------S----------L--------E--------------------------
    Bw47  --------F--------------------------------S------------------E--------------------------
    Bw65  ------W--------------N-F------------------S------------------E---------------H----------
    B14   ------W--------------N-F----------....----S------------------E---------------H----------
    B18   --------------------HD-S------------------S------------------E---------------H----------
    B40*  ------S-------------HN---------------------------------------E--------------------------
    Bw41  ----W---------------HN-----------------....----------------D-----------------D--E--
    Bw60  --------------------HN--------------------S---L--------------E-----------------DK-E--
    B8    ------S-------------HN---------------------------------------D-----------------D--E--
    Bw42  ------S-------------HN---------------------------------------D-----------------D--E--
    B7.1  ------S-------------HD--------------------------------E---R-----E-----------------DK-E--
    B7.2  ------S-------------HD-X------------------------------E---R-----E-----------------DK-E--
    Cw1   ------W-C---L--------D-----------------------------------E---R--------------------S----
    Cw2.1 ------------L--------D-S-----------------------------E---W-----E-----------------K----
    Cw2.2 ------------L--------D-S-----------------------------E---W-----E--------------------
    Cw3   ---II---------------D-H-------------------N-------------E----------L--------K------G-
consensus GSHTLQRMYGCDVGPDGRLLRGYHQYAYDGKDYIALNEDLRSWTAADTAAQITQRKWEAARVAEQLRAYLEGTCVEWLRRYLENGKETLQRA
             100        110        120        130        140        150        160        170        180
```

Figure 1.4(a) continued.

cleft. This implies that allelic polymorphisms are functionally important and are likely to result in differences in HLA class I-restricted immune responses (see later chapters). Two points have emerged from the comparison of allelic sequences: (1) multiple amino-acid differences are found between alleles, but alleles at the same locus are more similar to one another than to alleles of another locus; and (2) substitution of even a few amino acids is sufficient to alter serological and T-cell recognition. For example, HLA-A*0201 and HLA-A*6901 differ at only six amino-acid residues in the α1 domain, yet they are distinguishable by serology and by allospecific T-cells. The differences between HLA-A and HLA-B molecules are more numerous, for example, HLA-A*0201 and HLA-B*2701 differ by 14 amino acids over the α1 and α2 domains. Furthermore, the amino-acid sequences of the relatively non-polymorphic α3 and transmembrane domains differ significantly between the three "isotypes" of class I molecules (Parham et al., 1989b). From these comparisons, it has been possible to predict where serological epitopes lie in the linear sequence of the molecule, and these predictions have subsequently been verified by mutagenesis experiments (Salter et al., 1987). Sequence comparisons also provide a basis for α3 domain

```
              190       200       210       220       230       240       250       260       270
consensus DPPKTHVTHHPISDHEATLRCWALGFYPAEITLTWQRDGEDQTQDTELVETRPAGDRTFQKWAAVVVPSGEEQRYTCHVQHEGLPKPLTLRW
    A2.1  -A----M---AV------------S------------------------------G-------------Q---------------------
    A2.2Y -A----M---AV------------S------------------------------G-------------Q---------------------
    A2.2F -A----M---AV------------S------------------------------G-------------Q---------------------
    A2.3  -A----M---AV------------S------------------------------G-------------Q---------------------
    A2.4a -A----M---AV------------S------------------------------G-------------Q---------------------
    A2.4b -A----M---AV------------S------------------------------G-------------Q---------------------
    Aw69  -A----M---AV------------S------------------------------G-------------Q---------------------
    Aw68.2 -A----M---AV------------S------------------------------G-----V------Q---------------------
    Aw68.1 -A----M---AV------------S------------------------------G-----V------Q---------------------
    A3.1  ------M----------------------------------------------G-------------------------------------
    A3.2  ------M----------------------------------------------G-------------------------------------
    A11   ------M----------------------------------------------G-------------------------------------
    A1    ------M----------------------------------------------G-------------------------------------
    A32   -A----M---AV------------S------------------------------G-----S-----Q---------------------
    Aw24  ------M----------------------------------------------G-------------------------------------
    Bw58  ----------V--------------------------------------------------------------------------------
    B27.1 ------------------------------------------------------------------------------------------
    B27.2 ------------------------------------------------------------------------------------------
    B27.3 ------------------------------------------------------------------------------------------
    B27.4 ------------------------------------------------------------------------------------------
    B27f  ------------------------------------------------------------------------------------------
    B44.1 ------------------------S-----------------------------------------------------------------
    B44.2 -------------------V----------------------------------------------------------------------
    B13   ------------------------------------------------------------------------------------------
    Bw47  ------------------------------------------------------------------------------------------
    Bw65  ------------------------------------------------------------------------------------------
    B14   ------------------------------------------------------------------------------------------
    B18   ------------------------------------------------------------------------------------------
    B40*  ------------------------------------------------------------------------------------------
    Bw41  ------------------------------------------------------------------------------------------
    Bw60  ------------------------------------------------------------------------------------------
    B8    ------------------------------------------------------------------------------------------
    Bw42  ------------------------------------------------------------------------------------------
    B7.1  ------------------------------------------------------------------------------------------
    B7.2  ------------------------------------------------------------------------------------------
    Cw1   EH--------V-----------------------W------------------G-------M-----------------------E----
    Cw2.1 EH--------V---------------T-------------------------G-------------------------------E----
    Cw2.2 EH--------V---------------T-------------------------G-------------------------------E----
    Cw3   EH--------V-----------------------W-----------------G-------------------------------E----
consensus DPPKTHVTHHPISDHEATLRCWALGFYPAEITLTWQRDGEDQTQDTELVETRPAGDRTFQKWAAVVVPSGEEQRYTCHVQHEGLPKPLTLRW
              190       200       210       220       230       240       250       260       270
```

Figure 1.4(a) continued.

understanding the structural variations in subtypes of common alleles such as HLA-A2 and HLA-B27. Ten different HLA-A2 sequence subtypes and six different HLA-B27 alleles are now recognized (WHO Nomenclature Committee, 1990). The subtypes differ from one another by 1–5 amino-acid substitutions in the α1 and α2 domains, usually in positions around the binding-cleft (Parham et al., 1989a). The fact that these discrete changes are detected by antibody and/or cellular techniques indicate that they are at sites of the molecule which are either accessible and/or of functional importance.

Two fundamental questions raised by the extensive polymorphism of HLA molecules are: how was the polymorphism generated, and why does it exist? From the comparison of DNA sequences, it is possible to determine the distribution and frequency of nucleotide substitutions that result in an amino-acid change (replacement substitutions), and nucleotide substitutions that do not cause an amino-acid change (silent substitutions). The α1 and α2 domains have a preponderance of replacement substitutions, whereas the majority of substitutions in the α3 domain are silent (Hughes and Nei, 1988). This implies that variation in the amino-acid sequences

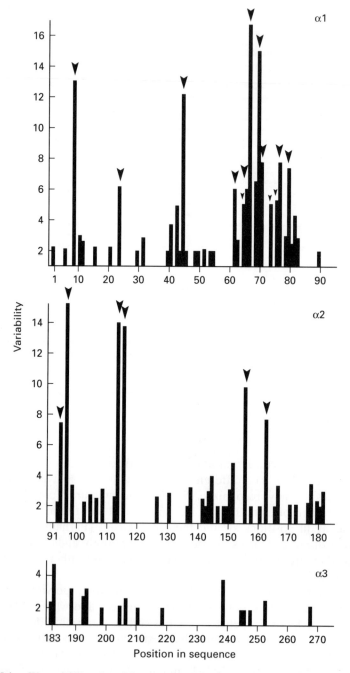

Figure 1.4 (b) Kabat–Wu variability plot of the same 39 HLA class I sequences. Separate plots of the three domains are shown. Variability is defined as the number of different amino acids found at a particular position divided by the frequency of the most common amino acid.

of the antigen-binding portion of the molecule is selected for in evolution, probably because it confers a functional advantage in terms of generating immune response differences (Chapter 3). The number of class I alleles in man makes it possible to generate effective immune responses against a wide variety of foreign antigens.

Various genetic mechanisms are likely to be involved in generating allelic diversity. Nucleotide substitutions or point mutations form the basis of diversity. From sequence comparisons of human and chimpanzee class I genes, it is apparent that the majority of these mutations are very ancient, and originated before divergence of human and chimpanzee lines some 3.3 million years ago. This argues against a special hypermutational mechanism in the generation of MHC diversity. Some alleles appear to be composed of segments from other allelic class I genes, leading to a patchwork motif of sequences shared with other alleles. This is likely to be the result of genetic recombination between alleles of the same locus, leading to segmental exchange of DNA sequences. A mechanism of non-reciprocal genetic exchange (gene conversion) has been invoked as the explanation for mutants of the murine H-2K^b gene (Nathenson et al., 1986); but this mechanism does not appear to be predominant in generating HLA class I diversity. Whatever the genetic mechanisms that generate diversity are, selection pressure remains the most important factor in fixing these polymorphic variations in a population.

Expression of class I genes

HLA class I molecules are found on most somatic cells in man, although the level of expression varies from tissue to tissue. They are not detectable on villous trophoblast, central nervous system neurones, corneal endothelium, and the exocrine portion of the pancreas; and only at low levels in endocrine tissue, myocardium, and skeletal muscle (Daar et al., 1984a). Variation in the expression of specific HLA alleles has also been reported. For example, some class I molecules are present in soluble form, and it has been observed that the level of HLA-A9 in serum is greater than that of other alleles (Botto et al., 1990). These allelic differences are due to differences in the gene structure.

The distribution of expression of the non-classical class I antigens differs from that of classical class I antigens (Table 1.3), but has been difficult to study due to a shortage of antibodies specific for these molecules. Sequencing of the HLA-E, HLA-F, and HLA-G genes showed that they were normal transcription units which encode a class I-like polypeptide. Furthermore, when HLA-G was transfected into a classical class I antigen-negative B-cell, it produced a molecule that was recognized by the monoclonal antibody W6/32 (which recognizes a non-polymorphic determinant on classical class I antigens) (Orr, 1989). HLA-G expression has been found in a choriocarcinoma cell line and in human chorionic cytotrophoblast cell membranes (Ellis et al., 1986, 1990), although these tissues do not express the classical class I antigens. A low amount of HLA-E RNA was detected in B-lymphoblastoid cells, a renal carcinoma cell line and a T-cell line, while higher levels were found in resting peripheral T-cells (Koller et al., 1988). The functional significance of non-classical class I gene expression is at present unclear.

Regulation of class I gene expression

The expression of class I molecules can be influenced both positively and negatively by many factors. Inflammatory mediators such as interferons, lymphokines, and cytokines increase expression of MHC class I products, and transformation of epithelial cells by viruses such as Adenovirus 12 leads to decreased levels of class I expression (Andersson et al., 1985). Given the role of MHC class I molecules in the presentation of endogenous antigens, a virus-induced decrease in class I antigen expression may provide a mechanism for the virus to escape the host's immune system; in contrast, increased levels of class I expression may facilitate virus eradication. Increased expression of a protein at the cell surface can be due to multiple mechanisms such as increased transcription of mRNA, increased mRNA stability inside the cell, and changes in the rate of processing of mRNA following transcription. In the case of class I molecules, increased expression is usually accompanied by an increase in the amount of mRNA.

The 5′ end of a eukaryotic gene usually contains the regulatory signals which direct gene transcription, such as enhancer and promoter sequences. The locations of some of the characterized regulatory elements of MHC class I genes are displayed in Figure 1.5. These regulatory elements may exert their effect in either a positive or negative manner. Analysis of the upstream sequences of murine and human class I genes has demonstrated the presence of several such enhancer sequences, which were identified by their ability to govern the in vitro expression of a reporter gene, chloramphenicol acetyltransferase (Kimura et al., 1986). Three important regions, located up to 550 bp upstream of the transcriptional start site of the murine H-2K^b gene have been localized, including one which is highly similar to the interferon response sequence found in a number of other human gene promoters (Friedman and Stark, 1985). These regions are capable of binding a number of DNA-binding proteins, which mediate the regulation of gene-transcription, and therefore sequence alterations in these regions can affect gene expression. Recently, a change of two nucleotides in the

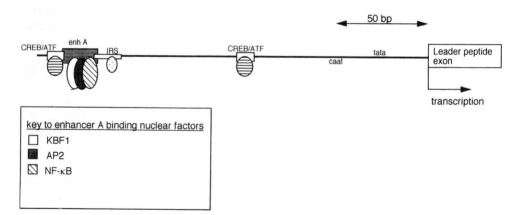

Figure 1.5 Regulation of transcription of class I genes. The location of the promoter sequences *tata* and *caat* are shown, as are the sequences which bind known transcription factors (boxes). The enhancer A (enh A) sequence binds multiple transcription factors. The CREB/ATF boxes represent the cAMP response elements, and probably bind proteins which belong to the CREB/ATF family. The interferon response sequence (IRS) binds several transcription factors (David-Watine et al., 1990).

promoter regions of the HLA-A3 and B7 genes have been found, and this change was sufficient to alter the level of expression (Hakem et al., 1989). Enhancer activity has also been demonstrated in the second intron of the human HLA-B7 gene, indicating that the regulation of class I transcription is complex, and is not mediated by one regulatory sequence alone (Ganguly et al., 1989).

Recent studies have characterized a number of transcription factors that are capable of binding to the five regulatory sequences present in the mouse K^b gene. The first to be identified was KBF1, which binds to the enhancer sequence A (Israel et al., 1987). The tissue distribution of KFB1 correlates well with the level of class I expression, and it has now been purified and shown to be a 48 kD protein (Yano et al., 1987). Of the other transcription factors, some bind specifically to the class I gene's regulatory sequences (such as KBF2 and H-2 transcription factor 1) and others (such as NF-κB and AP-2) can bind to regulatory sequences in other genes (David-Watine et al., 1990). Our current understanding is that multiple nuclear binding proteins are involved in the control of class I expression, and they interact with multiple regulatory sequences within the gene. Their identification and regulation is being actively pursued.

β2 Microglobulin (β2m)

Although the gene encoding this protein does not lie in the MHC (it is located on chromosome 15q21), β2m is non-covalently associated with all class I molecules, and constitutes the light chain. It was first isolated from the urine of patients with renal disease (Berggard and Bearn, 1968), and consists of 99 amino acids with a molecular weight of 11 800. In contrast to the HLA class I heavy chain, which is extremely polymorphic, there is no polymorphism of β2m in man. The protein sequence is highly conserved in mammalian evolution, and association of xenogeneic β2m with human class I molecules has been described. Indeed, a significant proportion of human β2m on human cells cultured in medium containing bovine serum is exchanged with bovine β2m supplied by the serum. The sequence of β2m shows strong homology to the constant region of immunoglobulin, the membrane-proximal domain of the class I heavy chain, and the class II α and β chains, making it a member of the 'immunoglobulin gene superfamily'. The structural homology to immunoglobulin was later confirmed by X-ray crystallography (Becker and Reeker, 1985).

Expression of β2 microglobulin

β2m is present on nearly all cell surfaces, and is also present in serum at a concentration of approximately 2 mg/l. The cellular synthesis and transport of β2m plays an important role in HLA class I expression, as demonstrated in the cell line Daudi (a Burkitt's lymphoma cell line), which fails to express HLA class I molecules on its cell surface due to an abnormal β2m mRNA (de Preval and Mach, 1983; Rosa et al., 1983). These data imply that β2m interacts with class I intracellularly, before transport to the cell surface. Recent experiments have shown that assembly of the class I heavy chain with β2m was not inhibited by the fungal antibiotic brefeldin A, which blocks the movement of newly synthesized membrane proteins from the endoplasmic reticulum (ER) to the Golgi apparatus. Therefore β2m and the class I heavy chain must associate within the ER, proximal to this site of blockade (Townsend et al., 1989). Once transported to the cell surface, β2m stays associated with the class I molecule, though it may be displaced by xenogeneic β2m as mentioned above.

From the crystallographic analysis of the class I structure, β2m and the α3 domain of the heavy chain are seen to be in the closest contact. However, α1 and α2 domains may also interact with β2m. When the HLA-B27 gene was transfected into mouse fibroblasts, it paired poorly with murine β2m, and expression was low when compared with a HLA-B7 transfectant. As the B27 and B7 molecules are identical in their α3 domain, the differences in β2m association can only be explained by differences in the α1 and α2 domains (Rein et al., 1987)

HLA class II genes

HLA-D region-encoded (or class II) molecules are heterodimeric membrane-bound glycoproteins which consist of an α (or heavy) chain of 35 kD, and a β (light) chain of 28 kD. The two chains are non-covalently associated. The amino-acid sequence of the two chains indicate that they each have two membrane-external domains of approximately 90 amino acids, and a transmembrane region and cytoplasmic domain of approximately 40 amino acids. The β chain contains two intrachain disulphide bonds, and the α chain a single intrachain disulphide bond. Cyrstallographic studies of HLA-DR1 showed that the structure of class II molecules is generally similar to that of class I, though the antigen-binding site has a more open conformation (Stern et al., 1993). The structure of class II molecules is represented schematically in Figure 1.2. Three separate isotypes of HLA-D region molecules are expressed – and have been named HLA-DR, DQ, and DP, respectively. The three molecules are encoded by genes located in distinct subregions of the HLA-D region itself (Figure 1.1), and exhibit different degrees of allelic polymorphism. Each subregion contains characteristic α and β chain genes, and their products assemble to give rise to the class II heterodimer. In addition to these expressed genes, other non-expressed, or only transiently expressed class II genes have been identified. In the current nomenclature, the protein product is denoted by α or β, and their respective genes by the suffix A or B. The HLA-DRα chain is therefore encoded by the HLA-DRA gene.

Gene organization of the HLA-D region

The entire HLA-D region spans approximately 1×10^6 bp, with the DP subregion located at the centromeric end, DR at the telomeric end, and DQ in between (Hardy et al., 1986). The gene structure of both A and B genes show the typical correspondence between functional domains and intron–exon structure as described for the class I genes, and portrayed in Figure 1.6. The α chain-encoding A gene consists of five exons, and the β chain-encoding B gene six exons (with the exception of DQB which has five) (Das et al., 1983; Larhammar et al., 1983; Okada et al., 1985; Spies

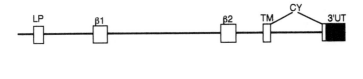

Figure 1.6 Genomic organization of HLA class II DQB gene (Larhammar et al., 1983). Exons are indicated in open boxes. LP=leader peptide; TM=transmembrane domain; CY=cytoplasmic domain; 3'UT=3'-untranslated sequence.

et al., 1985). Class II genes from the different subregions have a similar α and β chain gene structure. The DR region contains multiple DRB genes, which are not present in all MHC haplotypes. Some of these DRB genes are pseudogenes and are not expressed. The number of DRB genes and their patterns of expression are illustrated in Figure 1.7.

Linkage disequilibrium and recombination

One of the reasons that serological analysis of the HLA-D region antigens has been complicated is the presence of linkage disequilibrium across the MHC as a whole, and particularly in the HLA-D region. Linkage disequilibrium refers to the observation that alleles at two different loci on the same chromosome occur together more frequently than would be expected by chance. When this occurs these two alleles are said to be in linkage disequilibrium. For example, in the Caucasoid population HLA-A1 and HLA-B8 occur with individual gene frequencies of 27.5% and 15.7%, respectively. The predicted frequency of these two alleles being present on the same haplotype[1] would therefore be 4.3% (0.275 × 0.157 × 100). In fact, the A1 B8 haplotype is found in 9.8% of the population (Svejgaard et al., 1975). Thus A1 and B8 are said to be in linkage disequilibrium in Caucasians. Linkage disequilibrium has been observed between class I, class II, and class III alleles, and their frequencies in different ethnic groups have been documented (Baur and Danilovs, 1980a). Within the HLA-D subregion, linkage disequilibrium between DR and DQ alleles is very strong. However, there is only a weak linkage between DR and DP alleles which suggest that a hotspot of recombination may exist between the DQ and DP subregions. There are several possible explanations for the finding of linkage disequilibrium in a population. First it is possible that certain alleles are held together because they offer a selective advantage to their bearers, and haplotypes with this combination of alleles have therefore been preserved. A second possible explanation for linkage disequilibrium is that there has not been sufficient time for equilibrium to be established because the populations which bear the ancestral haplotypes have only mixed a relatively short time ago. The third explanation is that recombination sites are not randomly distributed, and there is an uneven distribution of these sites on haplotypes. The first explanation is the most likely one, as calculations have shown that the time required for linkage equilibrium to be reached within the MHC is very brief, when considered in the time course of human evolution.

---

[1] Haplotype refers to two or more polymorphic gene loci that are located on the same chromosomal segment.

The third explanation may be a contributory factor for the maintenance of disequilibrium, as Dawkins et al. have shown that certain MHC haplotypes are extremely well conserved during primate evolution (Dawkins et al., 1989).

The DR subregion

There is one DRA and multiple DRB genes in the DR subregion. The DRA gene shows very little polymorphism, indeed only one amino-acid substitution has been found from the sequencing of multiple genes – a substitution of leucine for valine at position 217 (Lee et al., 1982; Das et al., 1983). RFLP differences in the gene are due to non-coding region differences which map to the 3' end of the gene (Erlich et al., 1984).

By contrast, the DRB genes are extremely polymorphic. There is variation in the number of DRB loci within the subregion, in the number of loci which are expressed, and the number of alleles at each individual locus (Figure 1.7). In DR1 and DRw8 haplotypes, only one DRB gene is expressed compared to two DRB genes in all other haplotypes. These different gene products can be differentiated by protein chemical, serological, and by cellular typing techniques. The techniques used to define HLA polymorphism are discussed in more detail in Chapter 6. To date, nine DRB loci have been described: DRB1–9, of which all but DRB1,3,4 and 5 are pseudogenes. The DRB1 gene is expressed in all haplotypes but the second expressed DRB locus differs according to the haplotype. For DR4, DR7, and DRw9 it is DRB4, for DR2 it is DRB5, and for the remainder, it is DRB3. At present there are 60 DRB1 alleles, four DRB3 alleles, one DRB4 allele, and four DRB5 alleles, as shown in Table 1.2 (Bodmer et al., 1992). The use of the polymerase chain reaction to amplify specific

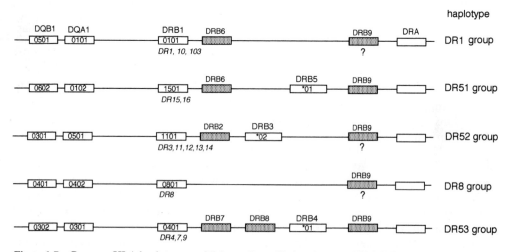

Figure 1.7 Common HLA haplotypes and linkage disequilibrium between HLA-DR and DQ alleles. The 1991 nomenclature of HLA alleles is used (Bodmer et al., 1992). The alleles of the DRB1, DQA1, and DQB1 loci are shown within the appropriate boxes. Shaded boxes indicate pseudogenes. The alleles of the other DRB loci which are expressed on different haplotypes are shown within the appropriate boxes. The question marks under the DRB9 genes on three haplotypes indicate that its presence on these haplotypes has to be confirmed.

DNA sequencies has greatly facilitated the analysis of HLA polymorphism and the structural basis of allelic variation (Saiki et al., 1988). On alignment of the allelic DRB sequences, it is apparent that substitutions are located in particular regions of the DRβ chain. Three regions of allelic hypervariability are clearly seen and are located around the peptide binding-site, in the floor and the wall of the groove, similar to the polymorphisms observed in class I molecules.

The polymorphisms of DRB gene structure and variation in the numbers of DRB genes on different haplotypes can also be detected by RFLP. Most HLA-D haplotypes show multiple hybridizing fragments (with the exception on DRw8 which only has one), and can be distinguished by their unique RFLP patterns. These patterns have been used to identify HLA-DR polymorphism for genotyping studies (Bidwell et al., 1988). Some DR haplotypes have similar RFLP patterns, such as DR3, DR5, and DRw6, which all express the DRw52 serological specificity from the DRB3 locus, and DR7 and DRw9, which express the DRw53 specificity encoded by the DRB4 locus. The similarities in these RFLP patterns are thought to reflect their shared evolutionary origins as they appear to have diverged from a common ancestral haplotype; this interpretation has been supported by other data obtained by pulse-field gel electrophoresis.

The DQ subregion

Two pairs of DQA and DQB genes are present in all haplotypes studied (Figure 1.1). The DQA1 and B1 genes are expressed and give rise to a well-characterized protein product. Although the DQA2 and B2 genes (previously also known as DX genes) are transcribed, no protein product from these loci has yet been defined. When DQ αβ dimers were first identified by alloantisera, they were referred to as DC molecules; DC was reclassified as DQ in 1984. In contrast to DR, there is polymorphism of both the DQA and DQB genes. By DNA sequence, 14 DQA and 19 DQB alleles have now been defined. As in the DRB genes, most of the allelic polymorphism resides in the membrane-distal α1 or β1 domains of the molecule, though they do not have the same discrete regions of allelic hypervariability as found in DRB genes (Bell et al., 1989).

As DQ polymorphism is in strong linkage disequilibrium with DR allelic variation, serological analysis of these antigens in the past gave supertypic reactivities, i.e. a polymorphism which is found in linkage with more than one HLA-DR allele. DR1, for example, is in linkage disequilibrium with the alleles DQA1*0101 and DQB1*0501 (previously recognized by antisera which were termed DQw1-specific), and DR5 with DQA1*0501 and DQB1*0301 (recognized by DQw3 antisera). Anti-DQw1 antisera also react with DR2 and DRw6 bearing cells, and anti-DQw3 antisera with DRw9 and a subset of DR4 bearing cells. Sequence and RFLP analysis of the DQA and DQB genes show an unusual relationship between their polymorphism and that of the DRB subregion. DQA polymorphism is strongly associated with DRB polymorphism at the RFLP and sequence level (Spielman et al., 1984; Moriuchi et al., 1985), while that of DQB is not so strongly linked, suggesting that recombinations may have occurred between DQA and DQB to generate some of the haplotypes present in the human population (Gregersen et al., 1988). The advent of PCR-based sequencing techniques allows more rapid study of DQ variation in different populations, and of the associations of DQ alleles with disease.

The DP subregion

There are two sets of HLA-DP genes within the subregion (Figure 1.1), although only the DPA1 and DPB1 genes are expressed as a product; the DPA2 and DPB2 genes are non-functional pseudogenes because of several deleterious mutations in the coding sequences (Servenius et al., 1984). Sequencing studies have revealed 38 DPB alleles, and the allelic variation seems to have arisen from a patchwork of sequence exchanges at specific positions within the DPB gene (Begovich et al., 1989). Although there is a large number of DPB alleles, they exhibit a lower level of amino-acid variation than that found in allelic DRB and DQB genes. At the DPA1 locus, eight alleles have been defined by sequencing. A listing of DP alleles is shown in Table 1.2. The considerable number of DPB alleles defined by DNA sequencing contrasts with the six alleles that were recognized previously by primed lymphocyte typing (PLT). A method of DP typing based on nucleotide sequence differences has been devised, using allele-specific oligonucleotide probes to hybridize to PCR-amplified DNA (Begovich et al., 1989). RFLP differences have also been demonstrated for the DPA and DPB genes, which show broad correspondence with DP typing by PLT (Bodmer et al., 1987; Hyldig-Nielsen et al., 1987), though they do not provide as detailed an analysis of polymorphism as the oligonucleotide method. As mentioned above, in contrast to DQ polymorphism, there does not appear to be strong linkage disequilibrium between DR and DP allelic variation.

HLA-DOB and HLA-DNA

The DOB gene was isolated from a cDNA library constructed from a B-lymphoblastoid cell line, and on sequencing showed approximately 70% nucleotide identity with DRB, DQB, and DPB genes. It is present in all haplotypes, and has been localized by pulse-field gel electrophoresis to the region between DQ and DP (Figure 1.1). Expression of this gene has only been detected at the mRNA level in B-cell lines, while T-cell lines and interferon-γ (γ-IFN)-treated fibroblasts gave no detectable signal (Tonelle et al., 1985).

The HLA-DNA gene (previously known as DZα or DOα) was first cloned from genomic DNA by hybridization with HLA-DRA. From its sequence, the gene appeared to be functional, but like HLA-DOB, only a weak signal was detected in Northern blots of B-cell RNA (Trowsdale and Kelly, 1985). The gene is located centromeric to HLA-DOB. Although it is tempting to speculate that the DNA and DOB gene products may pair to form a heterodimer, their asynchronous expression during B-cell differentiation argues against this possibility. No polypeptide for either chain has been detected to date.

HLA-DM

Two additional genes have recently been isolated and mapped to lie between HLA-DNA and DOB (Kelly et al., 1991). They have been termed DMA and DMB, respectively. Their sequences suggest that they are equally related to the known class I and class II genes, and may be early ancestors of the classical MHC genes of both the major classes. Modelling the structure of DM on the known structures of class I and class II molecules suggests that the DM molecule has a peptide-binding groove formed by the membrane-distal domains, but that this region of the molecule is more rigid than for other MHC molecules due to the presence of multiple cysteine residues that are likely to form intra-domain disulphide bonds. Their function is at present unknown, but they may present a limited set of peptides for immune recognition.

Expression of HLA-D region genes

In comparison with class I molecules, the range of tissue expression of class II molecules is much more limited (Daar et al., 1984a), but on induction by cytokines, this tissue range becomes extensive. Class II molecules are present constitutively on the cell surfaces of B lymphocytes, monocytes, macrophages, and dendritic cells, which all have the common property of being antigen-presenting cells for T lymphocytes. In addition, class II molecules are also found on vascular endothelium, various ductal epithelia (breast, gastrointestinal tract), and kidney glomeruli. This is summarized in Table 1.4.

Quantitative differences in the cell surface expression of DR, DQ, and DP are observed. DR is generally present in much greater quantities than DQ and DP. However, this pattern is not always found, and cell lines derived from lymphomas and leukaemias have been shown to express DP or DQ in the absence of DR (Symington et al., 1985; Lee, 1989).

Expression can be augmented or induced (in the case of class II-negative tissues) by cytokines and stimuli which activate cells (Table 1.5). The best studied is γ-IFN,

Table 1.4   Tissue distribution of HLA-DR antigen expression

Constitutive expression	Induced expression
Macrophage	Vascular endothelium
B cell	Gut epithelium
Dendritic cell	Dermal fibroblasts
Thymic epithelium	Melanocytes, astrocytes, Schwann cells, T-cells, thyroid follicular epithelium, synovial lining cells

Table 1.5   Influence of soluble factors on expression of HLA class II antigens

Factor	Effect
IFNγ	↑ in macrophages, fibroblasts, endothelium thyroid epithelium, etc. ↓ in B-cells
TNFα	↑ in macrophage, tumour cells
IL-4	↑ in B-cells, macrophages
IL-10	↑ in B-cells
LPS	↓ in B-cells, macrophages
PMA	↑ in B-cells
PGE2	↓ in B-cells, macrophages

LPS = lipopolysaccharide; PMA = phorbol myrstil acetate; PGE2 = prostaglandin E2; ↑ = increased expression; ↓ = decreased expression.

which has been shown to induce class II expression in fibroblasts, B-cell lines, T-cells, vascular endothelium, thymic epithelium and a range of other tissues (reviewed in Klareskog and Forsum, 1986). TNFα also increases class II expression on monocytes and macrophages, and it acts synergistically with γ-IFN (Arenzana-Seisdedos et al., 1988). The increase in surface expression is paralled by increases in the levels of mRNA transcription. The time course of this increase following stimulation of cells with γ-IFN has been well studied. DRA mRNA expression is maximal 2 days after exposure to γ-IFN, followed subsequently by DQ, for which maximal mRNA levels are reached after 4 days (Collins et al., 1984). The induction of expression of class II genes by cytokines may have some relevance to the pathogenesis of autoimmune disease and to the evolution of graft rejection, as histopathological studies have demonstrated aberrant expression of class II molecules in many sites of disease (Bottazzo et al., 1986). These include thyroid epithelium in Grave's disease, synovial lining cells in rheumatoid arthritis, biliary duct epithelium in primary biliary cirrhosis, and in renal allografts undergoing transplant rejection. Although the precise mechanisms for the induction of expression in these tissues have not been entirely worked out, γ-IFN is presumed to play an important role. The contribution of this aberrant expression of class II molecules, and consequent antigen presentation, to the pathogenesis and progression of autoimmune disease is discussed in Chapter 4.

Control of HLA class II gene expression

Transcriptional regulation of class II gene expression is mediated by a number of DNA-binding nuclear proteins which interact with control sequences at the 5′ end of the gene, regulating both tissue specific expression and induction of gene expression by cytokines. These control mechanisms have been studied at the molecular level using deletion constructs attached to reporter genes (Dorn et al., 1987; Sherman et al., 1989), gel retardation assays which detect DNA-binding regulatory proteins (Reith et al., 1989), and more recently, using transgenic mice which carry different deletion constructs of the H-2Ea gene (Le Meur et al., 1985; Pinkert et al., 1985; van Ewijk et al., 1988). Four different regulatory sequences (W, X, Y, and Oct) have been identified. They have distinct nucleic acid motifs, and are present at the 5′ end of the coding sequences of the murine class II genes Aa, Ea, and the human genes DRA, DQB and DPB, approximately 180 bp upstream of the initiation site of transcription (Benoist and Mathis, 1990) (Figure 1.8). Another control region, from 1000 to 2000 base pairs upstream of the transcription start site, also influences the cell type specificity of class II expression. Transgenic mice with 1.9 kb of the 5′ flanking sequences of the Ea gene show a correct pattern of class II expression in its tissues, but deletion of the 5′ flanking sequences down to 1.3 kb produced mice which expressed no Ea on their B-cells, yet Ea was present in the thymus, peripheral macrophages and dendritic cells (Yamamura et al., 1985; Widera et al., 1987; van Ewijk et al., 1988).

At least five B-lymphocyte nuclear proteins have been demonstrated to bind to the promoter regions of the DRA gene (Reith et al., 1989), and it is possible that even more regulatory factors will be found. These regulatory factors generally act in *trans*, that is they are not linked to the MHC genes themselves. This has been shown by gene complementation analysis of a class II negative B-cell line which was derived

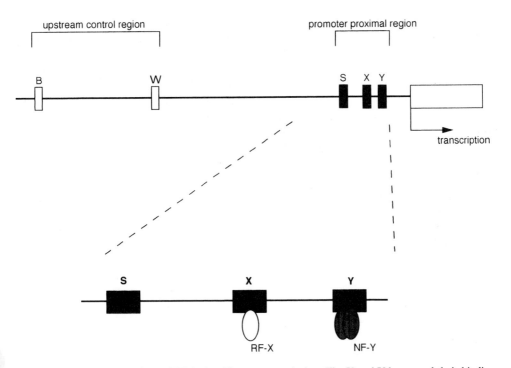

Figure 1.8 Regulatory regions of HLA class II gene transcription. The X and Y boxes and their binding to known transcription factors are shown. The O, W, and B (B-cell regulatory) regions have regulatory effects on class II transcription, but the factors that bind to these sequences are not known.

from the Burkitt lymphoma cell line RAJI by gamma irradiation. Fusion of this cell with murine B cells led to re-expression of its class II molecules, indicating that a factor provided by the murine cell can restore class II expression (Accolla et al., 1986). Other HLA class II-loss mutants with similar phenotypic properties have been described (Lee, 1989). In studies on a cell line derived from a patient with the bare lymphocyte syndrome – a rare form of severe combined immunodeficiency caused by a failure of HLA class II expression, lack of a *trans*-acting factor was also demonstrated (de Preval et al., 1985). One of these nuclear factors: RF-X, binds to the X-regulatory sequence, and is absent in lymphocytes obtained from the patient (Reith et al., 1988).

Proteins which bind to the Y and S sequences have been identified in a similar manner (Dorn et al., 1987; Tsang et al., 1990). From the experiments on the bare lymphocyte syndrome cells, it appears that the different *trans*-acting factors form a complex which is capable of regulating transcription, and that the lack of a single component is sufficient to abrogate transcription. The current state of knowledge about class II regulatory sequences and the factors that bind to these elements is reviewed by Glimcher and Kara (1992).

Class III genes

The class III region of the human MHC contains genes encoding the complement proteins C2, C4, and Factor B (Bf), as well as the gene for the cytochrome P-450 enzyme 21-hydroxylase (CYP21OH). There is extensive protein polymorphism for C4 and C2, while Bf and CYB21OH exhibit limited polymorphism. Physical mapping of the region has been achieved by a combination of cosmid cloning and pulse-field gel electrophoresis (Carroll et al., 1984; Dunham et al., 1987), and the orientation of the well-characterized genes are shown in Figure 1.9. The most centromeric genes within the region are those encoding steroid 21-hydroxylase (CYP21) and C4, which are tandemly duplicated in most haplotypes to give two pairs of genes: C4A and CYP21A, and C4B and CYP21B. The most telomeric is the gene for the complement component C2. Between C2 and HLA-B are the genes for tumour necrosis factor (TNFα and β) and for the heat-shock protein HSP70 (Spies et al., 1986). Recent studies of the DNA segment between C2 and HLA-B have revealed other transcribed sequences whose functions are as yet uncharacterized, and which appear to be highly conserved in evolution (Spies et al., 1989). It will be interesting to discover whether these new gene products play any role in immune recognition.

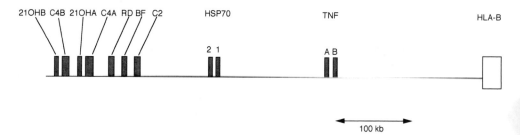

Figure 1.9   Genomic organization of the HLA class III region (Dunham et al., 1987; Sargent et al., 1989). 21OH = 21-hydroxylase; BF = Factor B; HSP70 = heat shock protein 70; TNF = tumour necrosis factor.

CYP21

Steroid 21-hydroxylase is a cytochrome P-450 enzyme of 494 amino-acid residues which hydroxylates progesterone at the 21 position in the synthetic pathway of cortisol. Deficiency of this enzyme results in the syndrome of congenital adrenal hyperplasia, which occurs in about 1/10 000 births. The CYP21B gene encodes the functional enzyme, while CYP21A is a pseudogene and is therefore not transcribed (Higashi et al., 1986). In classical 21-hydroxylase deficiency, 25% of the disease alleles result from a deletion spanning the CYP21B as well as the C4B gene, and the others appear to have resulted from gene conversion events which transposed deleterious mutations from the non-functional CYP21A gene to CYP21B gene (Globerman et al., 1988; Higashi et al., 1988).

C4

Both C4A and C4B are functional genes, which code for the fourth component of complement. This 200 kD serum protein is synthesized as a single precursor molecule which is then cleaved to form a mature protein with three chains α, β and γ, of 75, 95, and 30 kD, respectively. C4 participates in the classical pathway of complement activation; on cleavage of C4 by C1s, C4B complexes with C2 to form the active C3 convertase C4b2b. Two non-allelic electrophoretic variants of C4 are commonly present in serum, C4A (fast) and C4B (slow), encoded by the C4A and C4B genes, respectively. The two isotypes can also be distinguished by their reactions with Rodgers and Chido antisera, which react with C4d determinants present on the surface of the red blood cell (O'Neill et al., 1978). Functionally, C4A binds amine groups about 100 times more efficiently than C4B, while C4B binds hydroxyl groups more avidly (Law et al., 1984).

There are multiple alleles of each C4 locus, originally defined on the basis of electrophoretic mobility, including a null allele (absence of detectable protein) which is found in approximately 10% of C4A and 20% of C4B genes. Cloning and sequencing of the C4 genes has shown that the molecular basis of the difference between C4A and C4B resides in the α chain, in particular six amino acids within a stretch of 90 residues (Yu et al., 1986). Similarly, the molecular basis of the Rodgers and Chido reactivities has been elucidated. The amino-acid sequence Val, Asp, Leu, Leu (between amino acids 1188–1191 in the C4d region of the molecule) determines the Rodgers 1 epitope, while the sequence Ala, Asp, Leu, Arg at the same site determines Chido 1 reactivity (Yu and Campbell, 1987). In the Caucasoid population, C4A null alleles are most commonly due to deletion of a segment of the class III region which includes the C4A and CYP21A genes, and is readily detectable in RFLP studies (Carroll et al., 1985; Schneider et al., 1986). Null alleles are associated with a number of autoimmune diseases in man, the clearest example being systemic lupus erythematosus (Fielder et al., 1983; So et al., 1990). Complete C4 deficiency, as a result of homozygous deficiency of C4 at both loci, is rare, and is commonly associated with a systemic lupus erythematosus (SLE)-like illness (reviewed in Lachmann and Walport, 1987). However, establishing that disease susceptibility is conferred by the presence of a C4 null allele is complicated by the strong linkage disequilibrium between class I, class II, and class III genes, and diseases such as SLE are commonly associated with the inheritance of an MHC haplotype which includes A1, B8, and DR3 as well as a C4 null allele. This is discussed further in Chapter 9.

RD

This gene was initially identified in the mouse and subsequently its human homologue was identified (Levi-Strauss et al., 1988). It is located between Bf and C4, and nucleotide sequencing showed it to encode a novel polypeptide of 375 amino acids. It is unusual in that it lacks a hydrophobic leader sequence, and the gene is expressed in all tissues studied. The predicted peptide sequence has a region of 52 residues which consists of alternating basic and acidic amino acids such as arginine and aspartic acid, hence the name RD. The function of this protein is unknown.

Factor B (Bf) and C2

Factor B and C2 are members of the serine protease family of proteins, and play an important role in activation of the complement cascade. The main action of C2 is in the classical pathway of complement activation. On binding to C4b, C2 is cleaved into C2a (a fragment of Mr 70 kD) which remains complexed with C4b, and has C3 convertase activity. Factor B binds to activated C3 (C3i) in the presence of Factor D to form the alternative pathway C3 convertase C3bBb, which cleaves C3 to generate C3b. This complex also has C5 convertase activity.

Both proteins possess the typical serine protease domain at their C-termini, which has the characteristic triad of active site residues His, Asn, and Ser, at specific positions within the domain. This domain is also found in other serine proteases (such as elastase, trypsin, and chymotrypsin), and there is significant amino-acid homology over this region between them (Campbell and Bentley, 1985). The FB gene is 6 kb in size (Campbell and Porter 1983), and encodes a protein of 739 amino acids, and a Mr of 90 kD. Although C2 has a similar Mr to Factor B (Mr 102 kD), its gene is 18 kb in size (Bentley and Porter, 1984), due to the presence of larger introns. In common with other proteins which are capable of binding to C4b and C3b, such as C4 binding protein (C4BP) and β2-glycoprotein I, Factor B has three short consensus repeats (SCRs) of 60 amino acids each at its N-terminus, suggesting that the SCRs play a role in this interaction.

Both C2 and Bf are polymorphic, but the number of common alleles in the population (<5) is much lower than for C4 (Alper et al., 1972; Alper, 1976). C2C is the most common C2 allele, and F and S are the common Factor B alleles. There is limited RFLP of both genes (Woods et al., 1984; Bentley et al., 1985), and this genetic variation correlates with C2 and Factor B protein polymorphisms. Deficiency of C2 is rare, but it is the most prevalent genetic complement deficiency in man. The incidence of homozygous deficiency is 1 in 10 000 (Agnello, 1978) and a high proportion (approximately 40%) of these individuals have an SLE-like disease (Rynes, 1982). In the cases studied, the molecular basis appears not to be due to a major DNA deletion, but an inability to transcribe the mRNA (Ruddy, 1986). In contrast, total deficiency of Factor B has not been reported, suggesting that this condition may be lethal. Heterozygous deficiency states have been reported (Mauff et al., 1980; Tokunaga et al., 1984), but the molecular basis for them is unclear.

Tumour necrosis factor (TNFA and B)

Both these proteins are encoded by genes located between HLA-B and C2, about 600 kb centromeric to HLA-B (Spies et al., 1986). They are both expressed: TNFα as a mature protein of 156 amino acids and TNFβ as a protein of 171 amino acids. Both TNF genes have been cloned, and shown to share 35% amino-acid sequence homology (Gray et al., 1984; Pennica et al., 1984). Both are secreted from activated macrophages and activated T lymphocytes in the course of the inflammatory response, and have pleitropic actions on many cell types including other lymphocytes, neutrophils, and vascular endothelium (Ruddle, 1986; Kehrl et al., 1987). These effects include cytostatic and cytotoxic effects against certain tumour cell lines, induction of acute phase gene expression in hepatocytes (Perlmutter et al., 1986), and increased transcription of HLA class I molecules by vascular endothelium (Lapierre et al., 1988).

Heat shock protein 70

Two genes, 12 kb apart, encode two members of the 70 kD family of heat shock proteins (Sargent et al., 1989). They lie 92 kb telomeric to the C2 gene. Heat shock proteins have general functions in maintaining protein unfolding and intracellular trafficking of proteins, though the functions of the 70 kD proteins are not yet known.

Other genes within the MHC

The application of gene cloning techniques has uncovered a host of new genes within the MHC, particularly between HLA-B and the class III region and in the class II region. Intense interest has focused on the recently identified peptide transporter and proteasome genes, and how they influence the loading of MHC molecules with peptides in antigen presentation. The function of many of the other novel genes has yet to be defined. These newly discovered genes within the HLA region are discussed in more detail in Chapter 9.

Summary

Our understanding of the structure and complexity of the MHC region has grown as more powerful techniques to study the structure of the proteins, and the genes which encode these proteins, have become available. The number of currently identified genes within this region is approximately 50, and within the next few years, it is likely that all the genes within the MHC will be identified. However, the function of some of the recently cloned genes have yet to be elucidated, and it will be interesting to determine whether their location within the MHC relates to the immunological functions of the known class I, II and III gene products.

The detailed genetic map of the region, and our ability to distinguish polymorphisms at each of the loci within the MHC, will also enable us to determine the precise association between MHC polymorphisms and disease, and to answer the vexed question of whether an association with a particular HLA allele is really secondary to linkage of the HLA allele with an allele of another gene in close proximity. The identification of the 'disease susceptibility gene' will hopefully allow a clearer understanding of the mechanisms, and possible therapies for these diseases.

References

Accolla, R., Jotterand-Bellomo, M., Scarpellino, L. et al. (1986). Alr-1, a newly found locus on mouse chromosome 16 encoding a trans-acting factor for MHC class II gene expression. *J. Exp. Med.* **164**: 369–374.

Agnello, V. (1978). Complement deficiency states. *Medicine (Baltimore)* **57**: 1–23.

Alper, C.A. (1976). Inherited structural polymorphism in human C2: evidence for genetic linkage between C2 and Bf. *J. Exp. Med.* **144**: 1111–1115.

Alper, C.A., Boenisch, T. and Watson, L. (1972). Genetic polymorphism in human glycine rich beta-glycoprotein. *J. Exp. Med.* **135**: 68–80.

Anderson, M., Paabo, S., Nilsson, T. et al. (1985). Impaired intracellular transport of class I MHC antigens as a possible means for adenoviruses to evade immune surveillance. *Cell* **43**: 215–222.

Arenzana-Seisdedos, F., Mogensen, S.C., Vuillier, F. et al. (1988). Autocrine secretion of tumor necrosis factor under the influence of interferon-gamma amplifies HLA-DR gene induction in human monocytes. *Proc. Natl Acad. Sci. USA* **85**: 6087–6091.

Bach, F. and Hirschhorn, K. (1964). Lymphocyte interaction: a potential histocompatibility test in vitro. *Science* **143**: 813–814.

Baur, M.P. and Danilovs, J.A. (1980a). Reference tables for two and three locus haplotype frequencies of HLA-A, -B, -C, DR, Bf and GLO. In *Histocompatibility Testing 1980* (ed. P.I. Terasaki), pp. 994–1210, UCLA Tissue Typing Lab, Los Angeles.

Baur, M.P. and Danilovs, J.A. (1980b). Population analysis of HLA–A, B, C, DR and other genetic markers. In *Histocompatibility Testing 1980* (ed. P.I. Terasaki), pp. 955–993, UCLA Tissue Typing Lab, Los Angeles.

Becker, J.W. and Reeker, G.N., Jr (1985). Three dimensional structure of β2microglobulin. *Proc. Natl Acad. Sci. USA* **82**: 4225–4229.

Begovich, A.B., Bugawan, T.L., Nepom, B.S. et al. (1989). A specific HLA-DPβ allele is associated with pauciarticular juvenile rheumatoid arthritis but not adult rheumatoid arthritis. *Proc. Natl Acad. Sci. USA* **86**: 9489–9493.

Bell, J.I., Todd, J.A. and McDevitt, H.O. (1989). Molecular structure of human class II antigens. In *Immunobiology of HLA*, Vol. IIB (ed. B. Dupont), pp. 40–48, Springer-Verlag, New York.

Benoist, C.O. and Mathis, D.J. (1990). Regulation of major histocompatibility complex class-II genes: X, Y and other letters of the alphabet. *Ann. Rev. Immunol.* **8**: 681–715.

Bentley, D.R. and Porter, R.R. (1984). Isolation of cDNA clones for human complement component C2. *Proc. Natl Acad. Sci. USA* **81**: 1212–1215.

Bentley, D.R., Campbell, R.D. and Cross, S.J. (1985). DNA polymorphism of the C2 locus. *Immunogenetics* **22**: 377–390.

Berggard, I. and Bearn, A.G. (1968). Isolation and properties of a low molecular weight β2-globulin occuring in human biological fluids. *J. Biol. Chem.* **243**: 4095–4103.

Bidwell, J.L., Bidwell, E.A., Savage, D.A. et al. (1988). A DNA-RFLP typing system that positively identifies serologically well-defined and ill-defined HLA-DR and DQ alleles, including DRw10. *Transplantation* **45**: 640–646.

Bjorkman, P.J., Saper, M.A., Samraoui, B. et al. (1987). Structure of the human class I histocompatibility antigen, HLA-A2. *Nature* **329**: 506–512.

Bodmer, J., Bodmer, W.F., Heyes, J. et al. (1987). Identification of HLA-DP polymorphism with DPα and DPβ probes and monoclonal antibodies: correlation with primed lymphocyte typing. *Proc. Natl Acad. Sci. USA* **84**: 4596–4600.

Bodmer, J., Marsh, S.G.E., Parham, P. et al. (1990). Nomenclature for factors of the HLA system 1989. *Tissue Antigens* **35**: 1–8.

Bodmer, J., Marsh, S.G.E., Albert, E.D. et al. (1992). Nomenclature for factors of the HLA system 1991. *Eur. J. Immunogenetics* **19**: 327–344.

Bottazzo, G.F., Todd, I., Mirakian, R. et al. (1986). Organ-specific autoimmunity: a 1986 overview. *Immunol. Rev.* **94**: 137–169.

Botto, M., So, A.K., Giles, C.M. et al. (1990). HLA class I expression on erythrocytes and platelets with systemic lupus erythematosus rheumatoid arthritis and from normal subjects. *Br. J. Haematol.* **75**: 106–111.

Campbell, R.D. and Bentley, D.R. (1985). The structure and genetics of the C2 and Factor B genes. *Immunol. Rev.* **87**: 19–37.

Campbell, R.D. and Porter, R.R. (1983). Molecular cloning and characterization of the gene coding for human complement protein Factor B. *Proc. Natl Acad. Sci. USA* **80**: 4464–4468.

Carroll, M.C., Campbell, R.D., Bentley, D.R. et al. (1984). A molecular map of the human major histocompatibility complex class III region linking complement genes C4, C2 and Factor B. *Nature* **307**: 237–241.

Carrol, M.C., Palsdottir, A., Belt, K.T. et al. (1985). Deletion of complement C4 and steroid 21-hydroxylase genes in the HLA class III region. *EMBO J.* **4**: 2547–2552.

Collins, T., Korman, A.J., Wake, C.T. et al. (1984). Immune interferon activates multiple class II major histocompatibility complex genes and the associated invariant chain gene in human endothelial cells and dermal fibroblasts. *Proc. Natl Acad. Sci. USA* **81**: 4917–4921.

Daar, A.S., Fuggle, S.V., Fabre, J.W. et al. (1984a). The detailed distribution of HLA-A, B, C antigens in normal human organs. *Transplantation* **38**: 287–292.

Daar, A.S., Fuggle, S.V., Fabre, J.W. et al. (1984b). The detailed distribution of MHC class II antigens in normal human organs. *Transplantation* **38**: 293–298.

Das, H.K., Lawrence, S.K. and Weissman, S.M. (1983). Structure and nucleotide sequence of the heavy chain gene of HLA-DR. *Proc. Natl Acad. Sci. USA* **80**: 3543–3547.

Dausset, J. (1954). Leuco-agglutinins IV. Leuco-agglutinins and blood transfusion. *Vox Sang. (Amsterdam)* **4**: 190–198.

Dawkins, R.L., Kay, P.H., Martin, E. and Christinasen, F.T. (1989). The genomic structure of ancestral haplotypes revealed by pulsed field gel electrophoresis (PFGE). Immunology of HLA. In *Histocompatibility Testing 1987* (ed. B. Dupont), pp 893–895. Springer, New York.

David-Watine, B., Israel, A. and Kourilsky, P. (1990). The regulation and expression of MHC class I genes. *Immunol. Today* **11**: 286–292.

de Preval, C. and Mach, B. (1983). The absence of β2 microglobulin in Daudi cells: active gene but inactive messenger RNA. *Immunogenetics* **17**: 133–140.

de Preval, C., Lisowska-Grospierre, B., Loche, M. et al. (1985). A trans-acting class II regulatory gene unlinked to the MHC controls expression of HLA class II genes. *Nature* **318**: 291–293.

Dorn, A., Durand, B., Marfing, C. et al. (1987). Conserved major histocompatibility complex class II boxes – X and Y – are transcriptional control elements and specifically bind nuclear proteins. *Proc. Natl Acad. Sci. USA* **84**: 6249–6253.

Dunham, I., Sargent, C.A., Trowsdale, J. et al. (1987). Molecular mapping of the human major histocompatibility complex by pulsed-field gel electrophoresis. *Proc. Natl Acad. Sci USA* **84**: 7237–7241.

Ellis, S.A., Sargent, I.L., Redman, W.G. et al. (1986). Evidence for a novel HLA antigen found on human extravillous trophoblast and a choriocarcinoma cell line. *Immunology* **59**: 595–601.

Ellis, S.A., Palmer, M.S. and McMichael, A.J. (1990). Human trophoblast and the choriocarcinoma cell line BeWo express a truncated HLA class I molecule. *J. Immunol.* **144**: 731–735.

Erlich, H., Stetler, D., Sheng-Dong, R. et al. (1984). Analysis by molecular cloning of human class II genes. *Fed. Proc.* **43**: 3025–3030.

Fielder, A.H.L., Walport, M.J., Batchelor, J.R. et al. (1983). A family study of the MHC of patients with SLE. Null alleles of C4A and C4B may determine disease susceptibility. *Br. Med. J.* **286**: 425–478.

Friedman, R.L. and Stark, G.R. (1985). Alpha interferon induces transcription of HLA and metallothionein genes which have homologous upstream sequences. *Nature* **314**: 637–639.

Ganguly, S., Vasvada, H.A. and Weissman, S. (1989). Multiple enhancer-like sequences in the HLA-B7 gene. *Proc. Natl Acad. Sci. USA* **86**: 5247–5251.

Glimcher, L. and Kara, C. (1992). Sequences and factors: a guide to MHC class II transcrition. *Ann. Rev. Immunol.* **10**: 13–49.

Globerman, H., Amor, M., Parker, K.L. et al. (1988). A nonsense mutation causing steroid 21-hydroxylase deficiency. *J. Clin. Invest.* **82**: 139–144.

Gorer, P. (1936). The detection of antigenic differences in mouse erythrocytes by the employment of immune sera. *Br. J. Exp. Pathol.* **17**: 42–50.

Gray, P.W., Aggarwal, B.B., Benton, C.V. et al. (1984). Cloning and expression of cDNA for human lymphotoxin, a lymphokine with tumour necrosis activity. *Nature* **312**: 721–724.

Gregersen, P.K., Kao, H., Nunez-Roldan, A. et al. (1988). Recombination sites in the HLA class II region are haplotype dependent. *J. Immunol.* **141**: 1365–1368.

Hakem, R., Le Bouteiller, P., Barad, M. et al. (1989). IFN-mediated differential regulation of the expression of HLA-B7 and HLA-A3 class I genes. *J. Immunol.* **142**: 297–305.

Hardy, D.A., Bell, J.I., Long, E.O. et al. (1986). Mapping of the class II region of the human major histocompatibility complex by pulsed-field gel electrophoresis. *Nature* **323**: 453–455.

Higashi, Y., Tanae, A., Inoue, H. et al. (1988). Evidence for frequent gene conversion in the steroid 21-hydroxylase P-450 gene (C21) gene: implications for steroid 21-hydroxylase deficiency. *Am. J. Hum. Genet.* **42**: 17–25.

Higashi, Y., Yoshioka, H., Yamane, M. et al. (1986). Complete nucleotide sequence of two steroid 21-hydroxylase genes tandemly arranged in human chromosome: a pseudogene and a genuine gene. *Proc. Natl Acad. Sci. USA* **83**: 2841–2845.

Hughes, A.L., and Nei, M. (1988). Pattern of nucleotide substitution at major histocompatibility complex class I loci reveals overdominant selection. *Nature* **335**: 167–170.

Hyldig-Nielsen, J.J., Morling, N., Odum, N. et al. (1987). Restriction fragment length polymorphism of the HLA-DP subregion and correlation to HLA-DP phenotype. *Proc. Natl Acad. Sci. USA* **84**: 1644–1648.

Israel, A., Kimura, A., Kieran, M. et al. (1987). A common positive trans-acting factor binds to enhancer sequences in the promoters of mouse H-2 and β2-microglobulin genes. *Proc. Natl Acad. Sci. USA* **84**: 2653–2657.

Kehrl, J.H., Alvarez-Mon, M., Delsing, G.A. et al. (1987). Lymphotoxin is an important T cell-derived growth factor for human B cells. *Science* **238**: 1144–1146.

Kelly, A.P., Monaco, J.J., Cho, S. and Trowsdale, J. (1991). A new human-class II-related locus DM. *Nature*, **353**: 667–668.

Kimura, A., Israel, A., Le Bail, O. et al. (1986). Detailed analysis of the mouse H-2Kb promoter: enhancer-like sequences and their role in the regulation of class I gene expression. *Cell* **44**: 261–272.

Klareskog, L. and Forsum, U. (1986). Tissue distribution of class II antigens: presence on normal cells. In *HLA Class II Antigens* (ed. B. Solheim, E. Moller and S. Ferrone), pp. 339–348, Springer Verlag, New York.

Koller, B.H., Geraghty, D.E., Shimizu, Y. et al. (1988). HLA-E: a novel HLA class I gene expressed in resting T lymphocytes. *J. Immunol.* **141**: 897–904.

Koller, B.H., Geraghty, D.E., deMars, R. et al. (1989). Chromosomal organization of the human major histocompatibility complex class I gene family. *J. Exp. Med.* **169**: 469–480.

Lachmann, P.J. and Walport, M.J. (1987). Deficiency of the effector mechanisms of the immune response and autoimmunity. In *Ciba Foundation Symposium 129: Autoimmunity and Autoimmune Diseases* (ed. J. Whelan), pp. 149–171, Wiley, Chichester.

Lapierre, L.A., Fiers, W. and Pober, J.S. (1988). Three distinct classes of regulatory cytokines control endothelial cell MHC antigen expression. Interactions with immune gamma interferon differentiate the effects of tumor necrosis factor and lymphotoxin from those of leukocyte alpha and fibroblast beta interferons. *J. Exp. Med.* **167**: 794–804.

Larhammar, D., Hyldig-Nielsen, J. J., Servenius, B. et al. (1983). Exon–intron organization and complete nucleotide sequence of a human major histocompatibility antigen DCβ gene. *Proc. Natl Acad. Sci. USA* **80**: 7313–7317.

Law, S.K., Dodds, A.W. and Porter, R.R. (1984). A comparison of the properties of two classes, C4A and C4B, of the human complement component C4. *EMBO J.* **3**: 1819–1823.

Lawrance, S.K., Smith, C.L., Srivastava, R. et al. (1987). Megabase-scale mapping of the HLA gene complex by pulsed field gel electrophoresis. *Science* **235**: 1387–1390.

Lee, J. S. (1989). Regulation of HLA class II gene expression. In *Immunobiology of HLA*, Vol. II (ed. B. Dupont), pp. 49–61, Springer-Verlag, New York.

Lee, J., Trowsdale, J., Travers, P.J. et al. (1982). Sequence of an HLA-DR α-chain cDNA clone and intron–exon organization of the corresponding gene. *Nature* **299**: 750–752.

Le Meur, M., Gerlinger, P., Benoist, C. et al. (1985). Correcting an immune-response deficiency by creating Ea transgenic mice. *Nature* **316**: 38–42.

Levi-Strauss, M., Carroll, M.C., Steinmetz, M. et al. (1988). A previously undetected MHC gene with an unusual periodic structure. *Science* **240**: 201–204.

Mauff, G., Federmann, G. and Hauptmann, G. (1980). A Haemolytically inactive gene product of Factor B. *Immunobiol.* **158**: 96–100.

McDevitt, H.O., Deak, B., Shreffler, D. et al. (1972). Genetic control of the immune response. Mapping of the *Ir-1* locus. *J. Exp. Med.* **135**: 1259–1278.

Moriuchi, J., Moriuchi, T. and Silver, J. (1985). Nucleotide sequence of an HLA-DQα chain derived from a DRw9 cell line: genetic and evolutionary implication. *Proc. Natl Acad. Sci. USA* **82**: 3420–3424.

Nathenson, S.G., Geliebter, J., Pfaffenbach, G.M. et al. (1986). Murine major histocompatibility complex class-I mutants: molecular analysis and structure–function implications. *Ann. Rev. Immunol.* **4**: 471–502.

O'Neill, G.J., Yang, S.Y., Tegoli, J., Berger, R., Dupont, B. (1978) Chido and Rodgers blood group determinants are distinct antigenic components of human complement C4. *Nature* **273**: 668–670.

Orr, H.T. (1989). HLA class I gene family: characterization of genes encoding non-HLA-A, B, C proteins. In *Immunobiology of HLA*, Vol. II (ed. B. Dupont), pp. 33–39, Springer-Verlag, New York.

Parham, P., Lawlor, D.A., Salter, R.D. et al. (1989a). HLA-A, B, C: patterns of polymorphism in peptide-binding proteins. In *Immunobiology of HLA*, Vol. II (ed. B. Dupont), pp. 10–33, Springer-Verlag, New York.

Parham, P., Lawlor, D.A., Lomen, C.E. et al. (1989b). Diversity and diversification of HLA-A, B, C alleles. *J. Immunol.* **142**: 3937–3950.

Payne, R. and Rolfs, M.R. (1958). Fetal-maternal leucocyte incompatibility. *J. Clin. Invest.* **37**: 1756–1763.

Pennica, D., Nedwin, G.E., Hayflick, J.S. et al. (1984). Human tumour necrosis factor: precursor structure, expression and homology to lymphotoxin. *Nature* **312**: 724–729.

Perlmutter, D.H., Dinarello, C.A., Punsal, P.I. et al. (1986). Cachectin/tumor necrosis factor regulates hepatic acute-phase gene expression. *J. Clin. Invest.* **78**: 1349–1354.

Pinkert, C., Widera, G., Cowing, C. et al. (1985). Tissue-specific, inducible and functional expression of the Ead MHC class II gene in transgenic mice. *EMBO J.* **4**: 2225–2230.

Ploegh, H., Orr, H. and Strominger, J. (1980). Molecular cloning of a human histocompatibility antigen cDNA fragment. *Proc. Natl Acad. Sci. USA* **77**: 6081–6085.

Rein, R.S., Seeman, G.H.A., Neefjes, J.J. et al. (1987). Association with β2-microglobulin controls the expression of transfected human class I genes. *J. Immunol.* **138**: 1178–1183.

Reith, W., Satola, S., Herrero Sanchez, C. et al. (1988). Congenital immunodeficiency with a regulatory defect in MHC class II gene expression lacks a specific HLA-DR promoter binding protein, RF-X. *Cell* **53**: 897–906.

Reith, W., Barras, E., Satola, S. et al. (1989). Cloning of the major histocompatibility complex class II promoter binding protein affected in a hereditary defect in class II gene regulation. *Proc. Natl Acad. Sci. USA* **86**: 4200–4204.

Rosa, F., Fellous, M., Dron, M. et al. (1983). Presence of an abnormal beta2-microglobulin mRNA in Daudi cells. Induction by interferon. *Immunogenetics* **17**: 125–131.

Ruddle, N.H. (1986). Activation of human polymorphonuclear functions by interfon-gamma and tumour necrosis factor. *J. Immunol.* **136**: 2335–2336.

Ruddy, S. Component deficiencies. 3. The second component. (1986). *Prog. Allergy.* **39**: 250–266.

Rynes, R.I. (1982). Inherited complement deficiency states and SLE. *Clin. Rheum. Dis.* **8**: 29–47.

Saiki, R.K., Gelfand, D.H., Stoffel, S. et al. (1988). Primer-directed enzymatic amplification of DNA with a thermostable DNA polymerase. *Science* **239**: 487–491.

Salter, R.D., Clayberger, C., Lomen, C.E. et al. (1987). In vitro mutagenesis at a single residue introduces B and T cell epitopes into a class I HLA molecule. *J. Exp. Med.* **166**: 283–288.

Sargent, C.A., Dunham, I., Trowsdale, J. et al. (1989). Human major histocompatibility complex contains genes for the major heat shock protein HSP70. *Proc. Natl Acad. Sci. USA* **86**: 1968–1972.

Schneider, P.M., Carroll, M.C., Alper, C.A. et al. (1986). Polymorphism of the human complement C4 and steroid 21-hydroxylase genes. Restriction fragment length polymorphisms revealing structural deletions, homoduplications, and size variants. *J. Clin. Invest.* **78**: 650–657.

Servenius, B., Gustafsson, K., Widmark, E. et al. (1984). Molecular map of the human HLA-SB(HLA-DP) region and sequence of an SB-alpha(DP-alpha) pseudogene. *EMBO J.* **3**: 3209–3214.

Sherman, P.A., Basta, P.V., Moore, T.L. et al. (1989). Class II box consensus sequences in the HLA-DRA gene: transcriptional function and interaction with nuclear proteins. *Mol. Cell. Biol.* **9**: 50–56.

Snell, G. (1958). Histocompatibility genes of the mouse. II Production and analysis of isogenic resistant lines. *J. Natl Canc. Inst.* **21**: 843–877.

So, A.K.L., Fielder, A.H.L., Warner, C.A. et al. (1990). DNA polymorphism of major histocompatibility complex class II and class III genes in systemic lupus erythematosus. *Tissue Antigens* **35**: 144–147.

Spielman, R., Lee, J., Bodmer, W.F. et al. (1984). Six HLA-D region α-chain genes on human chromosome 6: Polymorphisms and associations of DCα-related sequences with DR types. *Proc. Natl Acad. Sci. USA* **81**: 3461–3465.

Spies, T., Morton, C.C., Nedospasov, S.A. et al. (1986). Genes for the tumor necrosis factors alpha and beta are linked to the human major histocompatibility complex. *Proc. Natl Acad. Sci. USA.* **83**: 8699–8702.

Spies, T., Blanck, G., Bresnahan, M. et al. (1989). A new cluster of genes within the human major histocompatibility complex. *Science* **243**: 214–217.

Svejgaard, A., Hauge, M., Jersild, C. et al. (1975). The HLA system. An introductory survey. *Monogr. Hum. Genet.* **7**: 1–100.

Symington, F.W., Levine, F., Braun, M. et al. (1985). Differential Ia antigen expression by autologous human erythroid and B lymphoblastoid cell lines. *J. Immunol.* **135**: 1026–1032.

Terhorst, C., Parham, P., Mann, D. et al. (1976). Structure of HLA antigens: amino acid and carbohydrate compositions and NH2-terminal sequences of four antigen preparations. *Proc. Natl Acad. Sci. USA* **73**: 910–914.

Tiwari, J.L. and Terasaki, P.I. (1985). *HLA and Disease Association*. Springer-Verlag, New York.

Tokunaga, K., Omoto, K., Yukiyama, Y. et al. (1984). Further study or a Bf silent allele. *Hum. Genet.* **67**: 449–451.

Tonnelle, C., deMars, R. and Long, E.O. (1985). DOβ: a new β chain gene in HLA-D with a distinct regulation of expression. *EMBO J.* **4**: 2839–2847.

Townsend, A.R.M., Ohlen, C., Bastin, J. et al. (1989). Association of class I major histocompatibility heavy and light chains induced by viral peptides. *Nature* **340**: 443–448.

Travers, P.J., Blundell, T.L., Sternberg, M.J.E. et al. (1984). Structural and evolutionary analysis of HLA-D-region products. *Nature* **310**: 235–238.

Trowsdale, J. and Kelly, A. (1985). The human HLA class II α chain gene DZα is distinct from genes in the DP, DQ and DR subregion. *EMBO J.* **4**: 2231–2237.

Tsang, S., Nakanishi, M. and Peterlin, B. (1990). Mutational analysis of the DRA promoter: cis-acting sequences and trans-acting factors. *Mol. Cell. Biol.* **10**: 711–719.

van Ewijk, W., Ron, Y., Monaco, J. et al. (1988). Compartmentalization of MHC class II gene expression in transgenic mice. *Cell* **53**: 357–370.

van Rood, J.J. (1962). Leucocyte grouping: a method and its application. Ph.D. thesis, Leiden University.

Ways, J.P., Coppin, H.L. and Parham, P. (1985). The complete primary structure of HLA-Bw58. *J. Biol. Chem.* **260**: 11924–11933.

WHO Nomenclature Committee (1990). Nomenclature for factors of the HLA system, 1989. *Immunogenetics* **31**: 131–140.

Widera, G., Burkly, L.C., Pinkert, C.A. et al. (1987). Transgenic mice selectively lacking MHC class II (I-E) antigen expression on B cells: an in vivo approach to investigate Ia gene function. *Cell* **51**: 175–187.

Woods, D.E., Edge, M.D. and Colten, H.R. (1984). Isolation of a complementary DNA clone for the human complement protein C2 and its use in the identification of a restriction fragment length polymorphism. *J. Clin. Invest.* **74**: 634–638.

Yamamura, K., Kikutani, H., Folsom, V. et al. (1985). Functional expression of a microinjected Eda gene in C57BL/6 transgenic mice. *Nature* **316**: 67–69.

Yano, O., Kanellopoulos, J., Kieran, M. et al. (1987). Purification of KBFI, a common factor binding to both H-2 and beta 2-microglobulin enhancers. *EMBO J.* **6**: 3317–3324.

Yu, C.Y., Belt, K.T., Giles, C.M. et al. (1986) Structural basis of the polymorphism of human complement components C4A and C4B: gene size, reactivity and antigenicity. *EMBO. J.* **5**: 2873–2881.

Yu, C.Y. and Campbell, R.D. (1987). Definitive RFLPs to distinguish between the human complement C4A/C4B isotypes and the major Rodgers/Chido determinants: application to the study of C4 null alleles. *Immunogenetics* **25**: 383–390.

Zinkerragel, R. and Doherty, P. (1974). Restriction of in vitro T cell-mediated cytoxicity in lymphocytic choriomeningitis within a syngeneic or semiallogeneic system. *Nature* **248**: 701–702.

CHAPTER 2

Structure and assembly of class I and class II molecules

Alex So

Department of Rheumatology
Royal Postgraduate Medical School
London, UK

Introduction

A detailed knowledge of the structure of HLA molecules is essential to our understanding of their functions in the immune response. Until the structure of the HLA-A2 molecule was solved by X-ray crystallography, our knowledge of the HLA molecule's structure was derived from a variety of analytical techniques. These included protein and nucleic acid sequencing, which provided the primary structure of the molecule and the nature of its allelic variations (see Chapter 1), and analysis of the consequences of naturally occurring and genetically engineered mutations of HLA molecules on antibody recognition and recognition by T cells. With the crystallization of HLA-A2, and the subsequent elucidation of its three-dimensional structure, we now have a detailed topographic map of the transplantation antigens. The structure of class II molecules has recently been solved crystallographically, and revealed that they share a very similar three-dimensional structure to that of class I molecules. The distinguishing feature of both class I and II molecules is the presence of a unique binding site for antigen which is formed by a floor of β-pleated sheets, and side walls of α-helices. This structure is elegantly tailored to fulfil the role of HLA molecules in antigen presentation, namely the binding of peptide fragments of antigen, and interaction with the T-cell antigen receptor. One important detail which emerged from the crystallographic studies is the observation that peptide fragments usually occupy this binding site, and this has led to a clearer understanding of how peptides and HLA molecules interact. Strong evidence for direct binding of peptide fragments to HLA molecules has been obtained in the past few years, and provides a structural explanation for the observed genetic differences in immune responsiveness, though other mechanisms affecting antigen processing and T-cell ontogeny also

HLA and Disease
ISBN 0–12–440320–4

(a)

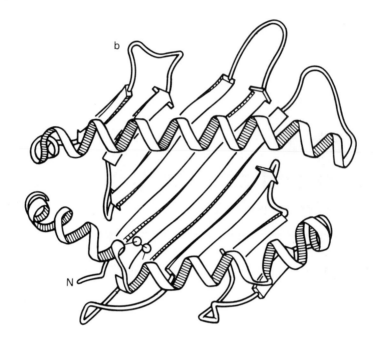

(b)

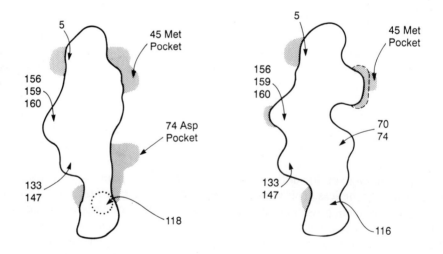

Figure 2.1 Schematic representation of the structure of HLA-A2 derived from crystallographic data (Bjorkman et al., 1987a, 1987b). (a) Ribbon diagram showing α-helices and β-pleated sheets. (b) Comparison of the peptide-binding pocket (left) with that of HLA-Aw68. Prominent pockets can be seen in Aw68 near positions 116 and 74. In A2 these pockets are filled by Arg at position 97 and Tyr at position 116, and by His at 74 (Garrett et al., 1989). A side view af HLA-A2 is shown in Plate I.

play a role in shaping the mature immune repertoire. This will be discussed in detail in Chapter 3.

The structure of HLA A-2

Bjorkman and colleagues published the detailed structure of the HLA-A2 molecule in 1987 (Bjorkman et al., 1987a, 1987b). A2 molecules were purified from a B-lymphoblastoid cell line JY, and subjected to papain digestion to remove the transmembrane anchor, and then immunopurified. X-Ray diffraction analysis was performed on the crystallized protein to 3.5Å resolution. The results showed that the molecule consists of two pairs of structurally similar domains: α1 and α2 have the same tertiary folding patterns, while α3 and β2m occupy a position proximal to the membrane and are composed of anti-parallel β-pleated sheets (Figure 2.1 and Plate I). The entire molecule is approximately 70Å in length, and at its membrane-distal portion, 50Å by 40Å across.

The antigen-binding site

The α1 and α2 domains each consists of four anti-parallel β-pleated sheets which are connected at their C-terminal ends to an α helix of approximately 35 amino acids. The helices are non-linear, and when viewed from the side, have an arched configuration. These two domains are paired so that the four β-pleated sheets from each domain form a single platform of eight β strands, and the α helices are separated from one another. The folded structure creates a groove which is 25Å by 10Å in size, and is the antigen-binding site of the HLA molecule. In the course of the X-ray crystallographic studies, it was observed that this groove consistently contained electron-dense material which was not accounted for by the polypeptide structure of the HLA molecule itself. This electron-dense material we now know to be peptide fragments within the binding site, which were co-purified with the HLA molecule.

Structural polymorphism of the antigen-binding site of class I molecules

When allelic sequences of the murine and human class I molecules were aligned to that of HLA-A2, the positions in the sequence which showed the greatest polymorphism were clustered around the antigen-binding site. Of the polymorphic amino-acid positions on HLA-A molecules, 15 out of 17 found on HLA-A2 were located in this area. The side chains of the amino acids found at the other two positions line small pockets which lie under the α helices, and contact the side chains of bound peptides. This lends support to the hypothesis that polymorphisms have been selected by their functional differences, based on their ability to present peptides to T lymphocytes. The crystallographic structure also enabled the identification of the possible contributions of particular amino-acid residues to peptide binding and/or contact with the

T-cell antigen receptor. Residues which are on the α-helical wall of the binding site have the potential to interact with both peptides and T-cell receptors, and those on the β-pleated sheet floor will predominantly interact with the peptide alone. This view correlates well with data on the effects on T-cell recognition of amino-acid substitutions (which occur naturally in allelic molecules, or were generated by site-directed mutagenesis) at these positions. Loss of T-cell recognition as a consequence of such substitutions implies that those positions are either involved in interaction with the peptide antigen, or with the T-cell receptor.

Crystallographic analyses have been performed on three allelic HLA class I molecules to date: HLA-A*0201 and HLA-A*6801, which differ by 11 amino acids at the polymorphic residues which contribute to the antigen-binding groove (Garrett et al., 1989), and HLA-B*2705 (Madden et al., 1991). Not surprisingly, all three molecules have a very similar overall structure. However, differences were seen in the shape of the peptide-binding site in all three alleles, in particular the conformation of pockets which contain polymorphic residues in the antigen-binding site. These pockets vary in shape and charge, and are capable of binding to a different array of peptide fragments. In HLA-A*6801, a deep negatively charged pocket, formed by the presence of Asp at position 74 (compared to His in HLA-A2), can be seen, and electron density representing peptide fragments can be seen to extend into this pocket. In the B27 molecule, peptide side chains make contact with pockets which are formed by positions 45, 74, 116, 152 and 156 of the HLA molecule. The HLA molecule can therefore determine the conformation of the bound peptide on the basis of these interactions, and particular peptide sequences may bind preferentially to individual HLA alleles. This hypothesis was confirmed by sequencing of peptide fragments eluted from murine and human class I molecules, and is discussed in more detail in a later section.

Assembly of class I molecules

The formation of the heterodimeric class I molecule takes place in the endoplasmic reticulum (ER), soon after translation of the class I heavy chain and the $\beta2$ microglobulin molecule. The molecule is then transported to the Golgi apparatus, where modifications to its glycosylation occur, followed by transport to the cell surface. We now know that peptide antigens, peptide transporter molecules and ATP-dependent processes all play important roles during this assembly process, and form the biochemical basis of the endogenous pathway of class I-restricted antigen presentation.

From experiments on a mutant murine cell line (RMA-S) which expresses very low levels of class I molecules, Townsend and his colleagues have established that the binding of endogenously derived peptides plays a vital role in the assembly and subsequent transport of class I heterodimers to the cell surface. One of the first observations to be made was that the RMA-S cell line was unable to display viral peptides for cytotoxic T-cell recognition when infected with live virus, but was efficiently lysed when pulsed with synthetic peptides that required no further processing. Biochemical studies revealed that the cells contained abundant amounts of class I heavy (α) and light ($\beta2m$) chains, but that these failed to give rise to stable

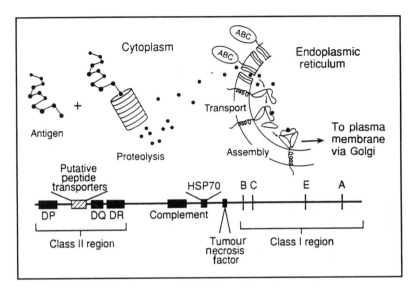

Figure 2.2   Proposed model of the structures and functions of the class I peptide transporters (TAP1 and TAP2) and the proteasome complex, together with their intracellular and genetic locations (taken from Parham, 1990). The degradation of cytoplasmic protein antigen into peptides (●), their transport into the endoplasmic reticulum and assembly with MHC class 1 molecules is shown. The location of the putative peptide transporter genes, and two genes that are thought to encode components of the proteasome complex within the class II region of the HLA complex is also illustrated.

complexes, and surface expression of the class I molecule is greatly reduced. They went on to show that normal levels of MHC class I expression could be achieved either by lowering the temperature of culture to 25°C, or by providing exogenous synthetic peptides which are able to bind to the cell's class I molecules (Townsend et al., 1989). On the basis of these and other results, it was postulated that these mutant cells were defective in the transport of endogenously derived peptide antigens from the cytosol into the ER, where class I assembly takes place, and that peptide binding plays a crucial role in the assembly of stable class I dimers. Under normal circumstances these molecules are unstable, and are degraded or internalized rapidly. However, they survive at low temperature and can be stabilized by the binding of added peptides. Similar lines of evidence, pointing to a gene within the MHC which regulates peptide transport, had been described previously on human mutant cell lines (DeMars et al., 1985; Salter and Cresswell, 1986). The identification of two peptide transporter genes (discussed in more detail in Chapters 3 and 9) within the MHC suggested that the molecules they encoded may be responsible for peptide entry into the ER (Figure 2.2). Transfection of the murine and human transporter genes into the mutant cell lines, such as RMA-S, restored normal levels of class I expression and antigen presentation ability, thus confirming that the defect in these variant cell lines is the absence of one or more of these transporter proteins (Powis et al., 1991; Kelly et al., 1992; Spies et al., 1992). When the assembly of class I molecules was studied in vitro, both peptide antigens and β2 microglobulin were shown to stabilize the conformation of the molecule (Townsend et al., 1990). It also became apparent that the assembly of class I molecules was an energy-dependent process and requires ATP

(Levy et al., 1991). It is possible that additional, as yet unidentified, proteins are required in the assembly step.

Site of interaction of class I antigens with CD8

In addition to interacting with peptide antigens and T-cell receptors, class I molecules also physically interact with the accessory molecule CD8. This interaction appears to increase cell:cell avidity and contribute to T-cell signalling. The α3 domain of the class I molecule has been shown to be the site of interaction with the CD8 molecule. Recently, the effects of site-directed mutations in the α3 domain of the HLA-A2 molecule on allospecific cytotoxicity and on CD8-mediated adhesion were studied systematically. The results showed that positions 223 to 229 in the α3 domain, situated on an exposed loop between strands 3 and 4 of the domain, appeared to be the major contact site for CD8. β Microglobulin has a similar loop region, although the contribution it makes, if any, to CD8 interaction is unclear at present (Salter et al., 1990).

Structure of class II molecules

The crystallographic structure of HLA-DR1 shows considerable similarities to that of class I molecules, and bears out the modelling studies which predicted that the two structures would be analogous (Brown et al., 1988). Class II molecules possess a similar antigen-binding site, formed by the association between the class II α1 and β1 domains; and allelic polymorphisms are predominantly in or around this site. Exon-shuffling experiments of the polymorphic β1 domains of murine class II molecules provided evidence that there is a close association between the NH2-terminal α1 and β1 domains, which is required for efficient pairing of the two component chains to form the mature molecule (Sant and Germain, 1989). However, the binding site differs from class I molecules in that it has a more open configuration at its ends, and may therefore accommodate longer peptides than the class I site. In support of this is the linear conformation of the peptide antigen bound to the DR1 crystal, which extends out of the binding site at both ends. The other major difference is that DR1 crystals are composed of αβ dimers, with the binding sites facing opposite directions. The significance of this last finding has yet to be established (Brown et al., 1993).

Structure of the peptide antigen

The evidence that T cells recognize peptide fragments associated with class I and class II molecules is reviewed in detail in Chapter 3. From analyses of antigen-specific T-cell clones, the minimal length of a peptide fragment which retains T-cell stimulatory properties can be deduced. For class I-restricted antigens, the minimum length is nine amino acids, while for class II-restricted antigens, the peptides vary in length, usually between 10 to 20 amino acids in length. Recently, the structural properties of a number of these peptide antigens have become clearer, as a result of crystallographic data and amino-acid sequencing of peptides eluted from MHC molecules (Table 2.1).

Table 2.1 Sequence motifs of peptides bound to HLA class I antigens

Class I	1	2	3	4	5	6	7	8	9
HLA-A2[a]	–	**L**	–	–	–	–	–	–	V
	–	M	–	E	–	V	–	K	–
	–	–	–	K	–	–	–	–	–
HLA-B27[b]	–	**R**	–	–	–	–	–	–	–
	R	–	–	–	–	–	–	–	K
	–	–	–	–	–	–	–	–	R
HLA-B53[c]	–	**P**	–	–	–	–	–	–	–
	–	–	–	E	I	–	–	–	–
HLA-B35[d]	–	**P**	–	–	–	–	–	–	Y
	–	–	F	–	–	–	–	–	–

Amino-acid sequence (single letter code) of eluted peptides from different HLA class I molecules, and the dominant motifs obtained by protein sequencing. The prevalence of particular amino acids in relation to their sequence position on the eluted peptides was determined ([a]Falk et al., 1991; [b]Jardetzky et al., 1991; [c]Hill et al., 1992). Dominant residues are indicated in bold, and commonly occurring residues indicated in italics.

Analysis of the crystallographic data obtained on HLA-B27 showed that the electron-dense material which occupies the antigen-binding site is made up of nonamers which are in an extended conformation, with a slight kink in the middle, between amino acids 3 and 4 (Madden et al., 1991). The N- and C-termini of the peptide probably play an anchoring role, by their proposed interactions with conserved amino acids (such as Tyr at positions 7 and 171, Lys at 146 and Thr at 143), which serve to bind the ends of the peptide to the class I molecule. The side chains protrude from the peptide backbone in a roughly alternating manner, such that some of them (positions 2, 3, 7 and 9) face inward to contact the HLA molecule, some (positions 5 and 6) are able to make contact with both the HLA molecule and the T-cell receptor, and others (positions 4 and 8) point towards the T-cell receptor. It is therefore not difficult to envisage allelic variations of the binding site altering the capacity of individual MHC molecules to interact with particular peptide sequences. The sequences of a number of naturally processed peptides have been determined by elution of peptides from HLA-B27, HLA-A2, and the murine class I molecules K^d, D^b and K^b using immunoaffinity purified class I molecules. This has revealed that different HLA alleles favour the binding of peptides with characteristic sequence motifs. For example, peptides which bind to HLA-B27 have in common Arg at position 2, and peptides eluted from D^b molecules have Asn at position 5. These dominant amino-acid residues have also been termed anchor residues, as they interact with the binding pockets in an allele-specific manner.

Information on the structure of peptides bound to class II molecules has not been as detailed. Peptides eluted from the murine class II molecules $H\text{-}2A^b$ and $H\text{-}2E^b$ were generally longer than class I-associated peptides, comprising between 13 and 17 amino acids. Unlike class I-peptides, no characteristic sequence motifs were noted for the set of peptides studied (Rudensky et al., 1991). However, when the peptide sequences of many different class II-restricted peptides were analysed, patterns of similarity have been suggested (Rothbard and Taylor, 1988; Sette et al., 1989). The role of key or anchor residues in class II-peptides have also not been clearly resolved. In one series of experiments, it was shown that most of the amino acids in a haemagglutinin peptide could be substituted by alanine, with the exception of one tyrosine residue, without affecting its binding to HLA-DR1 (Jardetzky et al., 1990). Key binding residues on the peptide antigen and the class II molecule may also be identified by sequential substitution of a known peptide sequence, to identify the effects of the substitutions on T-cell recognition (Allen et al., 1987; Rothbard et al., 1989a, 1989b).

There may well be differences between the rules governing the binding of peptide to class I and class II molecules, which relate to their structural differences.

Peptide binding to HLA molecules

T-cell recognition of antigen requires that peptide fragments become associated with MHC molecules. This step takes place in different cellular compartments, depending on whether the peptide is presented by a class I or a class II molecule (reviewed by Yewdell and Bennink, 1990; Brodsky and Gugliardi, 1991). The process of association of peptide with HLA molecules has been studied in vitro in a number of ways for class I and class II molecules. This has shown that (1) peptide binding to HLA molecules can be quantified; (2) the efficiency with which a peptide binds to an individual MHC molecule correlates, in most instances, with the use of that MHC molecule as a restriction element by T cells with specificity for the peptide in question; (3) at neutral pH, the kinetics of binding are slow: the rate of association between peptides and MHC class II molecules (K_a) has been calculated to be $\approx 1\text{M}^{-1}\text{s}^{-1}$, and

Table 2.2 Features of peptide binding by MHC class II molecules

Peptide	MHC	Association ($\text{M}^{-1}\text{s}^{-1}$)	Dissociation (s^{-1})	Affinity (K_d)	Reference
OVA 323–339	IA^d (pH7)	1.9	1.6×10^{-5}	2×10^{-6}M	Buus et al. (1986)
	IA^d (pH5)			0.76×10^{-6}M	Jensen (1991)
HA 307–319	DR1	120	1.6×10^{-6}	13×10^{-9}M	Roche et al. (1990)
PCC 88–104	IE^k	120	1.2×10^{-3}		Sadegh-Nasseri and McConnell (1989)
HEL 46–61	IA^k			2×10^{-6}M	Babbittet al. (1985)

OVA = ovalbumin; HA = influenza haemagglutinin; PCC = pigeon cytochrome c; HEL = hen egg lysozyme. For PCC, the kinetics of peptide association with MHC to form an intermediate complex is shown.

the dissociation rate is also slow (K_d) $\approx 3 \times 10^{-6}$ s^{-1}, with an overall low equilibrium constant of approximately 2×10^{-6} M (compared to the equilibrium constant of high affinity antibody–antigen binding, which is in the range of 10^{-9} to 10^{-10}); and (4) only a fraction of the available class II molecules are associated with the peptide: the proportion varies from 10 to 50%, depending on the assay used (Sadegh-Nasseri and McConnell, 1989).

Binding studies were first performed using purified class II molecules (Table 2.2). The binding of the peptide antigen can be assessed either using a radiolabelled peptide in gel filtration or equilibrium dialysis experiments, or using a photoreactive peptide analogue, so that binding can be assessed fluorometrically. Recently, flow cytometric detection of biotinylated peptides has also been used. As class II molecules associate with peptide predominantly in an endosomal compartment in an acidic environment, the rate of peptide association under these conditions has been studied. Maximal binding was observed between pH 4.5 to 5.5. The rate of association was markedly increased at pH 5 as compared to pH 7, and a decrease in the K_d was also observed at higher pH (Jensen, 1991). When living cells were used, the rate of association was rapid, and by 60 minutes, the reaction had reached equilibrium (Ceppillini et al., 1989). Similar results showing rapid binding to cell surface class II have been obtained using a variety of techniques (reviewed in Rothbard and Gefter, 1991). These findings agree well with the results of T-cell assays, in that antigen presenting cells pulsed with peptide antigen for as short a time as 60 minutes are able to present the peptide efficiently to T cells (Shimonkevitch and Colon, 1984). These assays make it possible to question whether known immune response differences between allelic HLA molecules are due to differences in peptide binding affinities, or due to differences in T-cell receptor recognition. The answer is that both probably play a part in governing immune responses. The early binding studies using ovalbumin and pigeon cytochrome-C peptides showed allelic differences in their binding to different H-2A molecules, which correlated with their known restriction (Babbitt et al., 1985; Buus et al., 1986). However, it was also observed that some peptide antigens can bind to a range of different class II alleles, although T-cell recognition of the peptide may not be observed with some of these MHC molecules (Roche and Cresswell, 1990a), indicating that the T-cell receptor specificities required to recognize certain MHC: peptide combinations may not be present in the T-cell repertoire. This is discussed further in Chapter 3.

Similar results have been obtained in binding of peptides to HLA class I molecules. There is allelic variation in the ability of different HLA-A and -B alleles to bind class I-restricted influenza peptides (Chen and Parham, 1989; Bouillot et al., 1989). In contrast to class II binding, only about 0.3% of the available pool of class I molecules bound peptide, much less than that found with class II molecules (10–50%, as described above). This may be because class I molecules associate with peptide antigen in a specific intracellular compartment which is not readily reproduced in vitro, or that once bound, the peptide/class I complex is much more stable, and therefore it may be more difficult to displace endogenous peptides co-purified with the class I molecule by addition of an exogenous peptide.

Assembly of class II–peptide complexes

The biochemistry of the MHC class II pathway of antigen presentation is still not completely understood. Following synthesis in the ER, the α and β chains of the class II molecule associate with the invariant (Ii) chain, a glycoprotein with a single transmembrane domain and an amino-terminal cytoplasmic tail (Figure 2.3). Three forms of the Ii chain with cytoplasmic domains of two different lengths are expressed as a result of alternate splicing and alternate translation initiation sites (Strubin et al., 1986; O'Sullivan et al., 1987), but whether they function differently is unknown. The α, β and Ii chain trimer exists intracellularly as a multimer of three trimers (Roche

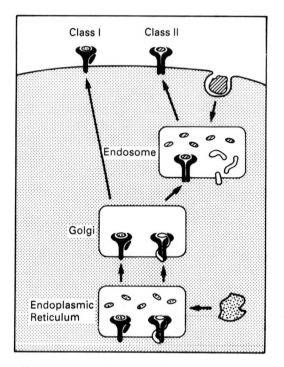

Figure 2.3   Intracellular traffic of MHC class I and class II molecules and antigen. MHC molecules are shown in black, the invariant chain in white, cytoplasmic antigen stippled, and endocytosed antigen hatched (taken from Long, 1989).

et al., 1991). Following glycosylation, the α, β and Ii trimer is transported to an endosomal compartment, where antigen processing takes place, and peptide antigens bind to the class II molecule. Direct evidence for the co-localization of all these molecules has been obtained by immuno-electron microscopy (Gugliardi et al., 1990). Two roles for the invariant chain has been proposed. First, it may have a role in preventing peptide occupancy of the class II binding site until it has reached the endosome. This was suggested by the observations that immature class II molecules which are still associated with Ii bind peptides much less efficiently than MHC class II dimers without associated Ii protein (Roche and Cresswell, 1990b), and that soluble constructs of the Ii chain inhibit peptide:class II association (Teyton et al., 1990). Second, it may provide signals for trafficking of the nascent class II molecule to the endosomal compartment. Evidence for this came from in vitro mutagenesis of the Ii chain. It was shown that amino acids 12–15 of the Ii chain are essential for intracellular transport to the endosome (Bakke and Dobberstein, 1990).

The processed antigen binds predominantly to newly synthesized class II molecules, though a proportion also binds to class II molecules which have been recycled from the cell surface (Reid and Watts, 1990; Davidson et al., 1991). The percentage of recycled class II has been estimated to be between 3 and 10% (Guagliardi et al., 1990; Neefjes et al., 1990).

The binding of peptide can also be accompanied by a conformational change in the class II heterodimer. Using purified class II molecules to bind peptide antigens at a variety of pH conditions, a floppy (F) form and a compact (C) form of the molecule were found. The C form can be distinguished from the F form by size, because it runs at a lower molecular weight (of 56 kD; cf. 63kD of the F form) (Dornmair et al., 1989). Experiments using metabolically labelled cells and purified class II molecules suggest that the C state is induced by peptide occupancy of the class II molecule, and imply that the F form may represent empty class II dimers, or dimers which have bound peptide in a different state (Germain and Hendrix, 1991; Sadegh-Nasseri and Germain, 1991). Studies of a naturally processed antigen bound to mouse H-2E^k molecules suggested that the initial binding of peptide to class II may take place in the F form (Srinivasan et al., 1991).

Summary

Much has been learnt about the structure and assembly of MHC molecules in the last 5 years. The interaction of these molecules with antigen, in particular the differing pathways of antigen processing, is still not completely characterized, and this will be a major area of research in the years to come.

Detailed knowledge of how peptides bind to MHC molecules may lead to novel ways of intervening in the antigen presentation pathway, which may be applicable in immunologically mediated diseases.

References

Allen, P.M., Matsueda, G.R., Evans, R.J. et al. (1987). Identification of the T-cell and Ia contact residues of a T-cell antigenic epitope. *Nature* **327**: 713–715.

Babbitt, B., Allen, P.M., Matsueda, G. et al. (1985). The binding of immunogenic peptides to Ia histocompatibility molecules. *Nature* **317**: 359–361.

Bakke, O. and Dobberstein, B. (1990). MHC class II-associated invariant chain contains a sorting signal for endosomal compartments. *Cell* **63**: 707–716.

Bjorkman, P.J., Saper, M.A., Samraoui, B. et al. (1987a). The foreign antigen binding site and T cell recognition regions of class I histocompatibility antigens. *Nature* **329**: 512–518.

Bjorkman, P.J., Saper, M.A., Samraoui, B. et al. (1987b). Structure of the human class I histocompatibility antigen, HLA-A2 *Nature.* **329**: 506–512.

Bouillot, M., Choppin, J., Cornille, F. et al. (1989). Physical association between MHC class I molecules and immunogenic peptides. *Nature* **339**: 473–475.

Brodsky, F.M. and Gugliardi, L. (1991). The cell biology of antigen processing and presentation. *Ann. Rev. Immunol.* **9**: 707–744.

Brown, J.H., Jardetzky, T., Saper, M.A. et al. (1988). A hypothetical model of the foreign antigen binding site of Class II histocompatibility molecules. *Nature* **332**: 845–850.

Brown, J.H., Jardetzky, T.S., Gorga, J.C. et al. (1993) Three-dimensional structure of the human class II histocompatibility antigen HLA-DR1. *Nature* **364**: 33–39.

Buus, S., Sette, A., Colon, S. et al. (1986). Isolation and characterisation of antigen-Ia complexes in T cell recognition. *Cell* **47**: 1071–1077.

Ceppillini, R., Frumento, G., Ferrara, G.B. et al. (1989). Binding of labelled influenza matrix peptide to HLA DR in living lymphoid cells. *Nature* **33**: 392–394.

Chen, B.P. and Parham, P. (1989). Direct binding of influenza peptides to class I HLA molecules. *Nature* **337**: 743–745.

Davidson, H.W., Reid, P.A., Lanzavecchia, A. et al. (1991). Processed antigen binds to newly synthesized MHC class II molecules in antigen-specific B lymphocytes. *Cell* **67**: 105–116.

DeMars, R., Rudersdorf, R., Chang, C. et al. (1985). Mutations that impair a posttranscriptional step in expression of HLA-A and -B antigens. *Proc. Natl Acad. Sci. USA* **82**: 8183–8187.

Dornmair, K., Rothenhausler, B. and McConnell, H.M. (1989). Structural intermediates in the reactions of antigenic peptides with MHC molecules. *Cold Spring Harbor Symp. Quant. Biol.* **54**: 409–416.

Falk, K., Rotzschke, O., Stevanovic, S. et al. (1991) Allele-specific motifs revealed by sequencing of self-peptides from MHC molecules. *Nature* **351**: 290–296.

Garrett, T.P.J., Saper, M.A., Bjorkman, P.J. et al. (1989). Specificity pockets for the side chains of peptide antigens in HLA-Aw68. *Nature* **342**: 692–695.

Germain, R.N. and Hendrix, L.R. (1991). MHC class II structure, occupancy and surface expression determined by post-endoplasmic reticulum antigen binding. *Nature* **353**: 134–139.

Guagliardi, L.E., Koppelman, B., Blum, J.S. et al. (1990). Co-localization of molecules involved in antigen processing and presentation in an early endocytic compartment. *Nature* **343**: 133–139.

Hill, A.V.S., Elvin, J., Willis, A.C. et al. (1992). Molecular analysis of the association of HLA-B53 and resistance to severe malaria. *Nature* **360**: 434–439.

Jardetzky, T., Gorga, J.C., Busch, R. et al. (1990). Peptide binding to HLA-DR1: a peptide with most residues substituted to alanine retains binding. *EMBO J.* **9**: 1797–1803.

Jardetzky, T.S., Lane, W.S., Robinson, R.A. et al. (1991). Identification of self peptides bound to purified HLA-B27. *Nature* **353**: 326–328.

Jensen, P.E. (1991). Enhanced binding of peptide antigen to purified class II major histocompatibility glycoproteins at acidic pH. *J. Exp. Med.* **174**: 1111–1120.

Kelly, A., Powis, S.H., Kerr, L.-A. et al. (1992). Assembly and function of the two ABC transporter proteins encoded in the human major histocompatibility complex. *Nature* **355**: 641–644.

Levy, F., Gabathuler, R., Larsson, R. et al. (1991). ATP is required for in vitro assembly of MHC class I antigens but not for transfer of peptides across the ER membrane. *Cell* **67**: 265–274.

Long, E. (1989). Intracellular traffic and antigen processing. *Immunol. Today* **10**: 232–234.

Madden, D.R., Gorga, J.C., Strominger, J.L. et al. (1991). The structure of HLA-B27 reveals nonamer self-peptides bound in an extended confirmation. *Nature* **353**: 321–325.

Neefjes, J.J., Stollorz, V., Peters, P.J. et al. (1990). The biosynthetic pathway of MHC class II but not class I molecules intersects the endocytic route. *Cell* **61**: 171–183.

O'Sullivan, D.M., Noonan, D. and Quaranta, V. (1987). Four Ia invariant chain forms derive from a single gene by alternate splicing and alternate initiation of transcription/translation. *J. Exp. Med.* **166**: 444–460.

Parham, P. (1990). Transporters of delight. *Nature* **348**: 674–675.

Powis, S.J., Townsend, A.R.M., Deverson, E.V. et al. (1991). Restoration of antigen presentation to the mutant cell line RMA-S by an MHC-linked transporter. *Nature* **354**: 528–531.

Reid, P.A. and Watts, C. (1990). Cycling of cell surface MHC glycoproteins cycle through primaquine sensitive intracellular compartments. *Nature* **346**: 655–657.

Roche, P. and Cresswell, P. (1990a). High affinity binding of an influenza haemagglutinin derived peptide to purified HLA-DR. *J. Immunol.* **144**: 1849–1856.

Roche, P. and Cresswell, P. (1990b). Invariant chain association with HLA-DR molecules inhibits immunogenic peptide binding. *Nature* **345**: 615–618.

Roche, P.A., Marks, M.S. and Cresswell, P. (1991). Formation of a nine-subunit complex by HLA class II glycoproteins and the invariant chain. *Nature* **35**: 392–394.

Rothbard, J. and Gefter, M.L. (1991). Interactions between immunogenic peptides and MHC proteins. *Annu. Rev. Immunol.* **9**: 527–565.

Rothbard, J. and Taylor, W.R. (1988). A sequence pattern common to T cell epitopes. *EMBO J.* **7**: 93–100.

Rothbard, J., Busch, R., Howland, K. et al. (1989a). Structural analysis of a peptide-HLA class II complex: identification of critical interactions for its formation and recognition by T cell receptor. *Int. Immunol.* **1**: 479–486.

Rothbard, J., Busch, R., Bal, V. et al. (1989b). Reversal of HLA restriction by a point mutation in an antigenic peptide. *Int. Immunol.* **1**: 487–494.

Rudensky, A.Y., Preston-Hurlburt, P., Hong, S.-C. et al. (1991). Sequence analysis of peptides bound to MHC class II molecules. *Nature* **353**: 622–627.

Sadegh-Nasseri, S. and Germain, R.N. (1991). A role for peptide in determining MHC class II structure. *Nature* **353**: 167–169.

Sadegh-Nasseri, S. and McConnell, H.M. (1989). A kinetic intermediate in the reaction of an antigenic peptide and I-Ek. *Nature* **337**: 274–276.

Salter, R.D. and Cresswell, P. (1986). Impaired assembly and transport of HLA-A and -B antigens in a mutant TxB cell hybrid. *EMBO J.* **5**: 943–949.

Salter, R.D., Benjamin, R.J., Wesley, P.K. et al. (1990). A binding site for the T-cell co-receptor CD8 on the alpha 3 domain of HLA-A2. *Nature* **345**: 41–46.

Sant, A.J. and Germain, R.N. (1989). Intracellular competition for component chains determines class II MHC cell surface phenotype. *Cell* **57**: 797–805.

Sette, A., Buus, S., Appella, E. et al. (1989). Prediction of major histocompatibility complex binding regions of protein antigens by sequence pattern analysis. *Proc. Natl Acad. Sci. USA* **86**: 3296–3300.

Shimonkevitz, R. and Colon, S. (1984). Antigen recognition by H-2 restricted T cells. *J. Immunol.* **133**: 2067–2074.

Spies, T., Cerundolo, V., Colonna, M. et al. (1992). Presentation of viral antigen by MHC class I molecules is dependent on a putative peptide transporter heterodimer. *Nature* **355**: 644–646.

Srinivasan, M., Marsh, E.W. and Pierce, S.K. (1991). Characterization of naturally processed antigen bound to major histocompatibility complex class II molecules. *Proc. Natl. Acad. Sci. USA* **88**: 7928–7932.

Strubin, M., Berte, C. and Mach, B. (1986). Alternative splicing and alternative initiation of translation explain the four forms of the Ia antigen-associated invariant chain. *EMBO J.* **5**: 3483–3488.

Teyton, L., O'Sullivan, D., Dickson, P.W. et al. (1990). Invariant chain distinguishes the exogenous and endogenous antigen presentation pathways. *Nature* **348**: 39–44.

Townsend, A.R.M., Ohlen, C. and Bastin, J. (1989). Association of class I major histocompatibility complex heavy and light chains induced by viral peptides. *Nature* **340**: 443–448.

Townsend, A., Elliot, T., Cerundolo, V. et al. (1990). Assembly of MHC class I molecules analyzed in vitro. *Cell* **62**: 285–295.

Yewdell, J.W. and Bennink, J.R. (1990). The binary logic of antigen processing and presentation to T cells. *Cell* **62**: 203–206.

CHAPTER 3

The roles of class I and II molecules of the major histocompatibility complex in T-cell immunity

Robert Lechler
Department of Immunology
Royal Postgraduate Medical School
London, UK

The context in which the products of the major histocompatibility complex were discovered accounts for their original naming as transplantation antigens. Observation of the phenomenon of allograft rejection led Peter Gorer to conclude that genetically determined differences, which he referred to as isoantigens, carried by the grafted tissue led to a vigorous immune response culminating in destruction of the foreign tissue (Gorer, 1938). Over the ensuing 40 years the physiological function of transplantation antigens has been elucidated, and it has become clear that they play a central role in specific immune responses. Their influence results from the fundamental requirement for T lymphocytes to recognize antigens only when complexed to an MHC molecule. Furthermore thymically expressed MHC molecules are responsible for selecting and shaping the mature T-cell repertoire. The extensive degree of polymorphism of MHC alleles within a species not only leads to differences in T-cell repertoire selection, but also leads to individual variation in immune responsiveness to many antigens. These aspects of the functions of MHC molecules will be addressed in turn in this chapter.

MHC restriction

The concept that antigen-reactive T-cells have specificity for both antigen and an MHC molecule arose from experiments carried out in guinea-pigs by Rosenthal and Shevach in 1973. They observed that T-cells from strain 2 guinea-pigs immunized in vivo against purified protein derivative (PPD) would only proliferate in vitro in response to PPD presented by peritoneal antigen-presenting cells (APC) from strain 2, and not from the MHC-incompatible strain 13, animals. In contrast, immune T-cells from strain $(2\times13)F_1$ animals would proliferate in response to APC from either parental strain. These results are summarized in Table 3.1. They further noted that, for the F_1 T-cells, alloantisera directed against the APC MHC type caused complete inhibition of the response. These results demonstrated that MHC products were acting as recognition elements for T-cells, and that T-cells exhibited allelic specificity for the co-recognized MHC molecule, a phenomenon that became known as MHC restriction.

Table 3.1   Demonstration of MHC restriction using antigen-presenting cells and T-cells from two inbred strains of guinea-pig

Antigen-presenting cell	T-cell	
	Strain 2	Strain 13
Strain 2	26 380	8 610
Strain 13	3 120	19 890

Animals were immunized in vivo with a preparation of mycobacterial antigen (PPD) and macrophages and T-cells harvested for in vitro rechallenge. The results of culturing the immune T-cells with PPD and macrophages from the histocompatible (MHC-matched) or histoincompatible (MHC-mismatched) strain are shown. Responses were measured as radioactive thymidine incorporation by dividing cells. Strong proliferation was only seen when the T-cells and the antigen-presenting macrophages were from the same strain, illustrating the phenomenon of MHC restriction (Rosenthal and Shevach, 1973).

Two major preoccupations in cellular immunology for the following decade were the molecular basis of MHC restriction, and the nature of the T-cell's antigen receptor. Some early models envisaged that T-cells were broadly self-MHC-restricted through one receptor(s) and carried an additional, separate antigen receptor. Using inbred mouse strains, including MHC recombinants, Zinkernagel and Doherty (1975) investigated the dual specificity of cytotoxic T-cells (CTL) specific for lymphocytic choriomeningitis virus, and restricted by either H-2K or H-2D MHC class I products. They found that, in order to compete for target cell lysis, it was necessary for viral and MHC antigens to be expressed on the same competitor cell, no competition occurred if virus-infected MHC-incompatible and uninfected MHC-compatible cells were added in excess. Two years later, Paul et al. (1977) showed, by in vitro manipulation, that two independent populations of T-cells existed in F_1 guinea-pigs, one restricted by each of the two parental MHC types. These observations suggested that there was a close linkage between the two specificities of a T-cell. One further indirect piece of evidence for the interdependence of recognition of the MHC restriction element and antigen was reported by Kappler et al. in 1981. Following the fusion of two murine T-cell hybridomas with specificity for MHC1 + x, and MHC2 + y, they were able to isolate fusion products that carried both of the parental reaction patterns, but they were unable to detect any cells that had a crossed specificity for MHC1 + y or for MHC2 + x. The strong implication of these data was that T-cells recognized a complex composed of an MHC molecule and an antigen, and that recognition occurred through a single receptor.

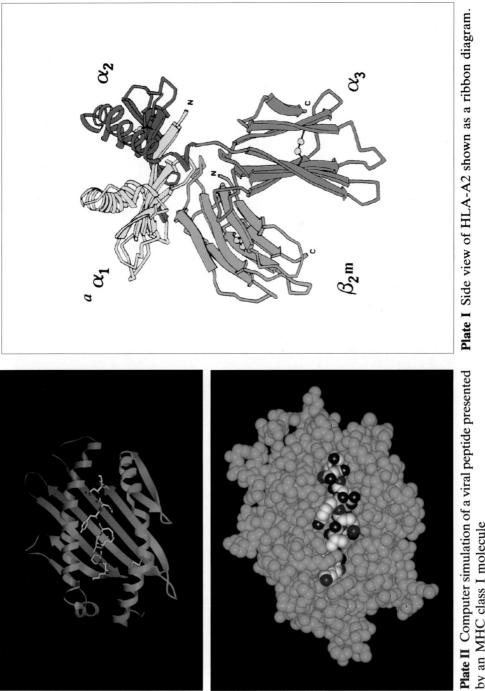

Plate I Side view of HLA-A2 shown as a ribbon diagram.

Plate II Computer simulation of a viral peptide presented by an MHC class I molecule

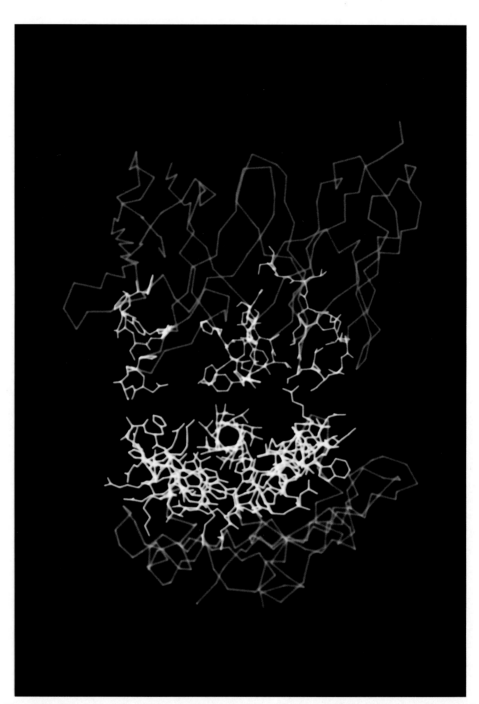

Plate III The tri-molecular complex of T-cell receptor, MHC molecule and peptide

The nature of antigen recognized by T-cells

It was thought at first that antigen bound to the surface of APC and was held there for T-cell recognition. When B cells were acting as the APC it was envisaged that the role of cell surface immunoglobulin was to bind and display antigen to T-cells, thereby forming an antigen bridge between the hapten-specific B-cell and the carrier-specific T-cell. Several groups, most notably Ziegler and Unanue (1981) provided evidence that a metabolically active step, requiring between 30 to 60 minutes, was required following the binding and uptake of soluble antigen by the APC. Treatment of the APC with aldehydes or with agents such as chloroquine that raise the pH of endocytic vesicles, either before antigen pulsing or within 30 minutes of antigen exposure, abolished antigen presentation. The nature of this processing step became clearer when it was noted that pre-fixed APC which were unable to present intact ovalbumin for T-cell recognition, could present a tryptic digest comprising peptide fragments of ovalbumin (Shimonkevitz et al., 1984). Since these observations were first made it has now become routine to define the specificity of a T-cell by using sets of short synthetic peptides derived from the antigen in question. In most cases the peptides that stimulate maximal T-cell responses are between eight and 20 amino acids in length, depending upon the class of MHC molecule to which the peptides are bound. It is reasonable to conclude from these observations that an important component of antigen processing by APC is the cleavage of internalized antigen into peptide fragments that are subsequently displayed for T-cell recognition.

As outlined in Chapter 2, these studies have been supplemented by the characterization of naturally processed peptides eluted from MHC class I (Falk et al., 1990; Jardetsky et al., 1991) and class II (Rudensky et al., 1991) molecules. These results have been obtained by acid elution of peptides from soluble MHC molecules purified from cell lysates, followed by high-pressure liquid chromatography (HPLC) separation of individual peaks of optical density. Material from these HPLC fractions have been subjected to microsequencing in order to determine the length of the peptides, and in some cases to define the protein from which the processed peptide was derived. Two important features of MHC class I-bound peptides have emerged from these results. First, the peptides that have been characterized are almost all nine amino acids in length. Peptides of this size would be readily accommodated as an open strand, in the MHC class I peptide-binding groove. Second, peptides isolated from an individual class I allele have conserved anchor residues at certain positions within the peptide sequence. For example, peptides eluted from the mouse class I molecule, H-2K^d, have a tyrosine residue at position 2, and most of the peptides have a hydrophobic residue at position 9 (Falk et al., 1990). In contrast, peptides eluted from the human class I molecule, HLA-A2.1, have either leucine or methionine at position 2, and valine or leucine at position 9. It is highly likely that the side chains of these anchor residues tuck into the allele-specific pockets that have been defined in the class I molecules whose three-dimensional structure has been solved by crystallographic techniques (Bjorkman et al., 1987; Garrett et al., 1989; Madden et al., 1991), as discussed in Chapter 2. A computer simulation of a viral peptide in the groove of a human MHC class I molecule is shown in Plate II.

Data regarding class II-bound peptides has been accumulating in recent months. The peptides that have been extracted from the mouse class II molecules, H-2A^b and H-2E^b, are significantly different from the class I-bound peptides described above.

Lengths between 13 and 17 amino acids have been observed, and no obvious consensus patterns have been detected (Rudensky et al., 1991). Two groups have characterized peptides eluted from HLA-DR1 molecules (Chicz et al., 1992; Hammer et al., 1992). Even more marked heterogeneity in size was noted, peptides ranging from 17 to 25 amino acids in length, with an average length of 15 residues. The semblance of a DR1-binding motif could be detected in this series of peptides, however, the interaction of peptides with class II molecules appears to be characterized by greater flexibility than is the case for class I molecules.

The need for proteolytic cleavage of antigen prior to class II-restricted T-cell recognition may not be true for all antigens or for all T-cells. For some hen egg lysosyme-specific T-cells, denaturation of the antigen is sufficient, and there appears to be no need for processing of any kind for T-cells reactive with the α chain of fibrinogen, a molecule which has no secondary structure (Lee et al., 1988). However, these are clear exceptions to a general set of rules, and almost certainly reflect the fact that the portions of these antigens seen by the T-cells in question are adequately displayed in the unfolded molecule, and that sufficient binding to the MHC restricting elements can occur without proteolytic cleavage.

MHC class discrimination in the presentation of antigens

All the early work on antigen processing and peptide recognition was confined to MHC class II-restricted responses. A short time later it became clear that the same principles applied to class I-restricted recognition of viral antigens (Townsend et al., 1985). A striking difference was noted, however, in that it was not possible to sensitize target cells for CTL-mediated lysis by the addition of soluble antigen. Class I-restricted presentation required either that the target cell was infected with the virus, or was transfected with the genes encoding the relevant viral protein. These latter findings suggested that presentation of antigen with a class I molecule requires that the antigen is synthesized inside the cell. Further evidence in support of this distinction between class I- and class II-restricted antigen presentation was provided by Morrison et al. (1986) who observed that exposure of cells to infectious virus led to antigen presentation with both class I and class II MHC products, but pulsing with killed virus was only able to induce class II-restricted presentation. They also noted that only the class II pathway was chloroquine sensitive. All these findings gave rise to the idea that two distinct routes of antigen processing and presentation exist, the class II pathway being favoured by the internalization of soluble antigen from outside the cell, or from the cell surface, and the class I pathway by the processing of antigens synthesized inside the cell (Germain, 1986).

The precise intracellular site at which proteins that are synthesized inside the cell become degraded into fragments for association with class I molecules has yet to be fully defined. Transfection of a truncated form of the influenza haemagglutinin gene that had no signal peptide-encoding sequence led to more efficient presentation than transfection of the intact gene including the signal sequence (Townsend et al., 1986). This implied that rapid entry into the endoplasmic reticulum (ER), as facilitated by the presence of an amino-terminal signal peptide, leads to impaired antigen process-ing, and that the ER is not the site of degradation. It is therefore assumed that peptides derived by proteolytic cleavage at another site, must be transported into the ER in order to meet and associate with nascent class I molecules. The recent cloning of genes, within the MHC regions of mice (Monaco et al., 1990), rats (Deverson et al., 1990), and humans (Spies et al., 1990; Trowsdale et al., 1990), which have homology to the family of multi-drug resistance genes, and which are predicted to have the function of transporting peptides into the ER, helps to fit one more piece into the jigsaw puzzle. The crucial role of these transporter genes, that appear to encode a dimeric complex composed of two proteins referred to as TAP1 and TAP2, is illustrated by the phenotype of mutant tumour cell lines that lack expression of one or other of the *TAP* genes. The mutant cells have very low levels of expression of class I molecules, and are unable to present virus-derived peptides for recognition by cytotoxic T-cells when infected with virus (Townsend et al., 1989). In contrast, these cell lines are perfectly able to present synthetic peptides for T-cell recognition. Furthermore, culturing the cells at low temperature (26°C) or in the presence of peptides that are known to bind to the cells' class I molecules leads to significant recovery of class I expression. The conclusion of all these studies is that, in the absence of an intact TAP complex, cells are unable to load class I molecules with peptides. Bound peptide makes such a major contribution to the assembly and stability of class I molecules, that in the absence of TAP proteins the class I molecules that reach the cell surface are limited to those that bind the small set of peptides that are generated in the ER by cleavage of signal peptides from proteins that are inserted into the ER (Engelhard et al., 1992), or travel to the cell surface 'empty'. The latter category of class I molecules are highly unstable at 37°C, but are more stable at 26°C, and can be stabilized by the addition of suitable peptides to the culture medium. These added peptides bind to the empty molecules as they reach the cell surface, and confer stability at that site.

Two additional genes in the same area of the class II region have also been cloned. These genes encode two components of proteasomes, which are multimeric complexes of low molecular weight proteins residing in the cytoplasm of all cells (Glynne et al., 1991). It is thought that proteasomes are the site at which proteins are degraded into peptides before being transported into the ER for loading on to class I molecules. The role of the two proteasome components that are encoded in the class II region is uncertain, in that the absence of expression of these genes does not have any obvious effect on the structure or function of class I molecules. Presumably these proteins have a more subtle effect that will emerge in time.

The major pathway of MHC class II peptide presentation has also become well-defined during the past few years. When class II αβ dimers form inside the cell, they associate in the ER with a third glycoprotein, the invariant chain (Ii). The Ii molecule is a non-polymorphic polypeptide with several molecular forms that are derived by alternative splicing of a single primary transcript. Four forms exist with molecular weights of approximately 33, 35, 41 and 43 kD. The significance of these different forms of the Ii molecule has not yet been fully resolved. The regulation of Ii expression in general parallels that of MHC class II products. The class II molecule remains complexed with the Ii chain until it reaches an endocytic compartment, where, under low pH conditions it dissociates from the Ii molecule, associates with peptide and is transported to the cell surface. There are two suggested roles for the Ii chain. One is to protect the class II molecule from peptide occupancy until it intersects the pathway of internalized exogenous antigen. This hypothesis is supported by the data of Roche and Cresswell (1990) who showed that the efficiency of class II:peptide association was 100-fold lower when the class II molecule was complexed with Ii. The same conclusion was drawn from the results of Teyton et al. (1990), who demonstrated that class II:peptide association could be inhibited by the addition of soluble Ii molecules. The alternative or additional function of the Ii molecule is to chaperone the class II molecule from the ER to the endosome, where peptide is available for binding and subsequent presentation (Bakke and Dobberstein, 1990; Teyton et al., 1990). These two roles for the Ii chain are not mutually exclusive, and both could be operative. It should be added that in transfection systems, it appears that the Ii molecule is required for the presentation of some (Stockinger et al., 1989), but not other (Peterson and Miller, 1990) exogenous antigens, although these experiments were conducted in a fibroblast cell line which does not present antigen with class II molecules under normal circumstances, and should therefore be interpreted with caution. Further information about the roles of the Ii chain has been provided by the recent generation of Ii- "knock-out" mice, in which the Ii gene has been silenced by the technique of homologous recombination. These mice have only 10% normal levels of expression of class II molecules at the cell surface, and are unable to make immune responses against many antigens (Viville et al., 1993; Bikoff et al., 1993). Despite these defects, the mice appear to be surprisingly healthy. It will require further study to elucidate the mechanisms whereby immune protection can be achieved under these circumstances.

As with most rules it is clear that exceptions do exist. The presentation of endogenous antigens with cell surface class II molecules has been described for several different antigens. For example, immunity to measles virus-infected cells, including cytotoxicity, is mainly class II-restricted. This may result from the manner in which measles virus particles fuse with cell membranes (Jacobson et al., 1989). In addition, Thomas et al. (1990) have shown that peptides of influenza haemagglutinin (HA) can be presented with cell surface class II molecules after transfection of class II-bearing cells with a truncated form of the HA gene which lacks a signal sequence. This HA molecule has no obvious means of reaching the cell surface or the endosomal compartment of the transfected cells. The same experiment has been conducted in human cells that lack an intact TAP complex. Absence of TAP expression made no difference to the presentation of the cytoplasmic HA protein to human T-cells, suggesting that class II molecules do not use the class I pathway even when cytoplasmic proteins are involved (Malnati et al., 1992). Similar findings have been reported following transfection of the gene encoding hen egg lysosyme (Moreno et al., 1991). However, it appears that even in these instances the loading of class II molecules with peptides may occur in the endosomal compartment of the cell. At this point there is no clear evidence that class II molecules can be loaded with peptide before reaching the endosome.

It has also proved to be possible to introduce exogenous antigen into the class I pathway artefactually, by allowing cells to internalize antigen under hypertonic conditions, and then subjecting the cells to a hypotonic shock causing lysis of pinosomes (Moore et al., 1988). The crucial event for class I-restricted presentation seems to be the delivery of antigen into the cytosol of the cell in order for antigen to enter the class I pathway. None the less, despite these apparent exceptions to the rule that class I and class II MHC molecules use two distinct pathways of antigen presentation, there does seem to be a strong bias for the presentation of internal, cytosolic proteins with class I, and external or membrane-bound protein with class II molecules. The features of the two major pathways of antigen presentation are summarized in Table 3.2. Class discrimination of this kind has an appealing logic to it, given that the large majority of CTL are class I-restricted. The consequence of this arrangement is that only virus-infected cells are lysed, and class II-bearing APC that internalize inactivated virus or viral products, and that are required for the generation of T-cell help, are protected from lysis by class I-restricted CTL. This has important implications for the presentation of autoantigens with MHC molecules of the two classes, as will be discussed later.

Table 3.2   Features of the antigen processing and presentation pathways associated with MHC class I and class II molecules

MHC class I pathway	MHC class II pathway
Peptides derived from cytoplasmic proteins	Peptides derived from extracellular and membrane-inserted proteins
Dependent on the actions of the TAP complex	Influenced by the invariant chain
Sensitive to Brefeldin A proteins	Requires synthesis of MHC class II
Insensitive to lysosomotropic agents such as chloroquine and NH_4Cl	Sensitive to lysosomotropic agents such as chloroquine and NH_4Cl
	Insensitive to Brefeldin A

It is worth emphasising, in this context, that most cell-surface MHC molecules are occupied with host-derived peptides all the time. The strongest evidence for this came from studies of a variant mouse B-cell line which had lost almost all its surface class I expression, due to a defect in peptide loading (Townsend et al., 1989; Ljunggren et al., 1990). This is described in detail above. Thus, only a tiny fraction of a cell's MHC molecules will be displaying an individual peptide at any one time.

The tri-molecular complex

The series of pieces of inferrential evidence of MHC:antigen association mentioned above were followed in 1985 by the direct demonstration of peptide binding to purified MHC molecules by equilibrium dialysis (Babbit et al., 1985). This report was followed by multiple other descriptions of the same observation using a series of different approaches. Furthermore, there were multiple instances in which a close correlation was seen between the efficiency of binding of a particular peptide to a particular MHC allelic product and the use of that MHC molecule as a restriction element for the peptide in question (Buus et al., 1987). These results established that the ligand specifically recognized by T-cells is a binary complex of MHC molecule and peptide.

At approximately the same time the major form of the T-cell's αβ antigen receptor was characterized biochemically (Samelson et al., 1983), and the genes encoding it were cloned from human (Saito et al., 1984; Yanagi et al., 1984) and murine (Chien et al., 1984; Hedrick et al., 1984) T-cells. Genetic analysis revealed that the T-cell receptor (TcR) genes, like their immunoglobulin counterparts, are rearranging genes, and generate diversity by an apparently random process of joining a variable (V), diversity (D) and junctional (J) segment to give rise to a functional expressible gene. The predicted three-dimensional structure of the T-cell receptor αβ dimer closely resembles that of a Fab fragment of an immunoglobulin molecule with a single major binding site formed by the interaction of the variable domains of the two chains (Davis and Bjorkman, 1988). A second dimeric T-cell receptor, γδ was defined subsequently on a small subpopulation of T-cells in the thymus and in the peripheral immune system (Brenner et al., 1986). In man, γδ-expressing T-cells represent approximately 5% of all peripheral T-cells. Whether or not the γδ receptor is MHC-restricted remains unclear, and the function of γδ-expressing T-cells has yet to be resolved. The best guess based on what is known of their distribution in the skin and the gut, and their specificity for conserved bacterial antigens, is that they provide an early and primitive form of defence at epithelial surfaces.

All the components of the tri-molecular complex that is at the heart of T-cell recognition had been defined in terms of primary sequence by 1985. The next major landmark was the definition of the three-dimensional (3-D) structure of the human MHC class I molecule HLA-A2 (Bjorkman et al., 1987), as discussed in detail in Chapter 2. This led to the proposal of a hypothetical model for class II structure that was supported by multiple independent lines of evidence. Very recently, crystallographic data has been obtained for HLA-DR molecules. The most striking finding as a result of analysing the class II crystals was the close similarity of the structures of class I and class II molecules. Subtle differences do exist, for example, the ends of the peptide-binding groove of the class II molecule are more open, consistent with the observation that class II-bound peptides can be substantially longer than those bound to class I molecules. None the less, the two structures are remarkably conserved. A model of the tri-molecular complex is represented schematically in Figure 3.1.

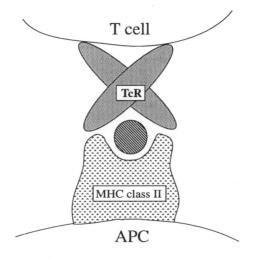

Figure 3.1   Schematic diagram of the tri-molecular complex. The three elements of the complex that is at the heart of T-cell recognition are shown, namely the dimeric T-cell receptor, an MHC molecule, and a bound peptide. The simultaneous interaction of the T-cell's receptor with the MHC molecule *and* with the MHC-bound peptide is illustrated.

One of the major points of debate about T-cell recognition hinges upon whether the T-cell's receptor has specificity for polymorphic regions of MHC molecules *and* for the MHC-bound antigen, or whether it has specificity for the antigen peptide alone. In the latter case, the phenomenon of MHC restriction has to be accounted for entirely by the influence of MHC polymorphism on which peptides are bound, and how they are orientated in the antigen-binding cleft for T-cell recognition.

The concept that two functionally distinct sites existed on MHC molecules was proposed in 1983 as the result of an extensive series of studies of cytochrome c-responsive T-cells (Heber-Katz et al., 1983). These two sites are illustrated diagrammatically in Figure 3.2. The upper surfaces of the two α helices form the T-cell receptor interaction site, referred to as the histotope because it confers *histo*compatibility. The inner aspects of the α helices together with the exposed portion of the floor of the groove form the peptide-binding surface, referred to as the desetope because the MHC molecule selects which determinants of an antigen will be presented, a phenomenon that has been called *determinant selection*. Within this model of MHC structure/function the TcR is envisaged to make specific contacts with amino-acid residues of the MHC-bound peptide, and with allele-specific residues on the histotopic surface of the MHC molecule. Several lines of evidence in support of this view have been described during the past few years:

(1) The location of allelically polymorphic residues on the upward pointing surface of class I and class II MHC molecules (Bjorkman et al., 1987; Brown et al., 1988). It is reasonable to assume that there has been selective evolutionary pressure that has preserved these polymorphisms, in order to ensure that the widest possible repertoire of TcR specificities is maintained in the population. If variation in these positions did not influence TcR recognition, it is difficult to understand why such variation would exist.

(2) The results of mutagenesis experiments in which residues in an MHC molecule that are predicted to be peptide-binding (desetopic) or TcR-contacting (histotopic)

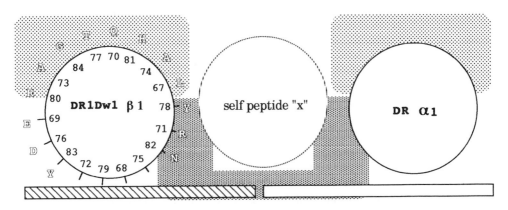

Figure 3.2   Two functional sites on MHC molecules involved in antigen recognition. The two amino-terminal domains of the human HLA class II molecule DR1Dw1 are represented schematically; the α helices are represented in cross-section with the amino acids located at positions 67–84 of the polymorphic β1 domain shown in single letter code, the platform of anti-parallel strands that compose the floor of the peptide-binding groove are represented as rectangles. The T-cell receptor-contacting (*histotopic*) surface is highlighted in light shading, and the peptide-binding (*desetopic*) surface in dark shading.

have been changed independently, and the mutated molecules tested functionally. The results of such experiments have implied an important role for residues in both of these locations on the MHC molecule (Ajitkumar et al., 1986; Ronchese et al., 1987; Barber et al., 1991).

(3) The frequent correlation between groups of MHC types which cross-react serologically and which are cross-reactively recognized by T-cells. Given that antibody epitopes have to be located on the exposed surfaces of MHC molecules in order to be available for binding, the fact that similar regions are responsible for serological and T-cell cross-reactions implies that the exposed portions of MHC molecules are involved in interactions with the TcR.

(4) The successful selection of thymocytes expressing a transgene-encoded TcR specific for antigen x + MHC y due to the presence in the thymus of MHC y alone, in the absence of x (Kisielow et al., 1988; Sha et al., 1988). Results of this kind imply that these transgene-encoded receptors have affinity for allele-specific features of the y MHC molecule itself.

An alternative view of T-cell recognition has been proposed by Claverie and Kourilsky (1986). Referred to as the peptidic self model, it envisages that all the specificity of the TcR is focused on the MHC-bound peptide, and little or no attention is paid to direct interactions with polymorphic residues on the MHC restricting element. There are two major points in favour of this view. The first is that only a small proportion of the allelically variable residues in the amino-terminal domains of MHC molecules are outside the peptide-binding site and available for TcR contact, 2–4 for class I and 3–5 for class II, compared to 12 or 13 that are predicted to interact with peptide. The second is that there appears to be no clear correlation between variable (V) region usage by T-cells and either the class, isotype or allele of MHC restriction element used by the T-cell. If an important component of the T-cell receptor's specificity is for polymorphic residues on the MHC molecule it would be predicted that there would be preferential usage of individual V segments by T-cells restricted by a particular MHC product. In answer to this point, it is possible that individual TcR molecules may be able to sit down on an MHC molecule in slightly different positions. In this case it is possible to envisage that several different TcR variable domains could interact in a specific manner with a single MHC product.

Although predictions can be made about the 3-D configuration of the tri-molecular complex, and about how the TcR sits on an MHC molecule (Davis and Bjorkman, 1988, and Plate III), until crystals of individual complexes are grown and analysed by X-ray diffraction these uncertainties will persist. One of the problems in discriminating between these possibilities is that it is difficult to rule out an influence by upward pointing residues on peptide binding, either due to a direct effect of their side chains, or by a distant conformational effect on the peptide-binding cleft. Furthermore, it is possible that the side chains of residues on the inner aspects of the α helices make contact with the TcR. The best compromise prediction that can be made with the currently available facts is that both models are true to a lesser or greater extent for individual T-cells. Given the apparently promiscuous use of V regions by T-cells it is likely that the affinity of a TcR for the MHC molecule it uses as a restriction element is low, none the less the maintenance of polymorphism in the genetic regions encoding the putative histotopic surface must have a reason, and implies that allele-specific contacts do contribute to the specificity of T-cell recognition.

The roles of CD4 and CD8

It has been known for several years that a close correlation exists between the CD4/8 phenotype of a T-cell and the class of MHC molecule by which it is restricted. Almost without exception CD4$^+$ T-cells are class II-restricted (Dialynas et al., 1983; Lo and Sprent, 1986) and CD8$^+$ T-cells class I-restricted (Swain, 1981). Direct evidence that the ligand for these T-cell surface molecules is the MHC molecule itself, of the appropriate class, was described for CD4 by Doyle and Strominger (1987), and for CD8 by Salter et al. (1990). The most recent observations about the function of these so-called accessory molecules suggest that they form an additional member of the molecular complex described above. Immobilized antibodies directed against the TcR cause T-cell activation, anti-CD4/8 antibodies alone do not. However, if T-cells were treated with conjugates of anti-TcR and anti-CD4/8 antibodies, that lead to cross-linking of the two molecules, the activating efficiency of the anti-TcR reagent was greatly augmented (Eichman et al., 1987). This synergy was only observed when the two antibodies were physically coupled, and no effect was seen of adding the anti-CD4/8 antibody separately. Furthermore, it appears that the CD4 molecule is physically coupled, in some way, to the TcR complex in the T-cell's membrane, in that the two molecules co-aggregate on the same surface of the cell (Kupfer et al., 1987). The contribution of CD4 ligation to the process of T-cell activation was made more clear by the discovery that the intracytoplasmic domains of CD4 and CD8 are non-covalently associated with a tyrosine kinase, p56^{lck} (Veillette et al., 1988). It appears that the interaction between CD4/8 and the class II/I molecule leads to the activation of this kinase and the subsequent phosphorylation of the ε chain of the CD3 complex.

The site on the MHC class I molecule with which CD8 interacts has been mapped

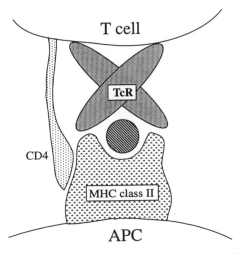

Figure 3.3 Schematic representation of the quaternary molecular complex. The CD4 T-cell co-receptor is shown interacting with the same MHC class II molecule as the T-cell's antigen receptor, at a site distant from the peptide-binding and TcR contact sites on the MHC molecule.

using naturally occurring (Salter et al., 1990) and in vitro-generated (Potter et al., 1989) mutants of human class I genes. The key residues are located in the membrane-proximal α3 domain on the class I heavy chain, residues 223–229 playing a dominant role.

The site on class II molecules with which CD4 interacts has been determined by a series of approaches, and maps to the β2 domain of the class II structure, parallelling the CD8:class I interaction (Lombardi et al., 1991; Cammarota et al., 1992; König et al., 1992). The concept of the tri-molecular complex still stands, in that it comprises the three elements that confer specificity on T-cell recognition, however, CD4 or CD8 represent a fourth member of the same physical complex and this four-member complex is portrayed in Figure 3.3.

Influence of MHC molecules on the expressed T-cell repertoire

As mentioned at the start of this chapter, the allelic polymorphism of MHC molecules is reflected in extensive variation in immune responsiveness to individual antigenic determinants, according to the inherited MHC genotype. There are many mechanisms underlying these immune response (Ir) gene effects, all of which have obvious potential relevance to HLA and disease associations, as discussed in Chapters 5 and 7. In order to understand these mechanisms it is important first to discuss the influence of thymically expressed MHC products on the selection of the mature T-cell repertoire. It appears that during the process of thymocyte ontogeny, differentiating thymocytes are subjected to positive and negative selective pressures, as discussed below.

Positive selection

The first requirement of the T-cell repertoire is that all the TcRs expressed on T-cells exported from the thymus are able to recognize antigen in association with MHC molecules, since all αβ-expressing T-cells only recognize antigen when it is physically complexed with an MHC molecule. Whether or not this requires an active selection process depends upon whether the germline encoded variable segments of TcR molecules have evolved to have intrinsic affinity for MHC products. Certainly it would be very uneconomical if this were not the case, and it appears that all the Vα and Vβ genes that are represented in the germline can be utilized by peripheral T-cells that have undergone thymic selection, albeit with widely varying frequencies. Also in favour of germline bias towards the MHC of the species is the fact that TcR Vβ genes show little capacity to cross-hybridize across species barriers (Patten et al., 1984) implying that TcR genes are largely species-specific. The second constraint on the T-cell repertoire is that it should be composed of T-cells that are capable of utilizing the particular MHC alleles possessed by the host, giving rise to the phenomenon of MHC restriction. In addressing this issue, the results of a large series of murine bone marrow chimaera and/or thymus allograft experiments conducted between the mid-1970s and the mid-1980s suggested that thymocytes are selected for recognition of thymic MHC polymorphisms. The general design of these experiments involved the injection of MHC heterozygous (A × B) bone marrow stem cells into leucocyte-depleted parental strain A or B strain mice, or the transplantation of an A or B strain thymus into an athymic (A × B)F_1 recipient animal. The F_1 T-cells of these animals, following differentiation in an A or B strain thymus was found to be strongly biased towards the thymic MHC type (Fink and Bevan, 1978; Zinkernagel et al., 1978; Lo and Sprent, 1986). The recent results of Marrack et al. (1988) supplement these chimaera models. They observed that thymocytes from H-2$^{b × k}$ mice treated from birth with monoclonal antibodies (mAbs) directed against either the class II molecules of H-2^b or H-2^k, when transferred into irradiated recipients of either the b or k haplotype together with antigen, gave rise to antigen-specific responses strongly biased to the untreated MHC class II type. This last experiment avoids the complexities of chimaeras and further supports the concept that MHC alleles expressed in the thymus are responsible for the selection of receptors with specificity for the thymic MHC types. The most persuasive evidence for intra-thymic positive selection of the repertoire is provided by transgenic mouse models, in which rearranged TcR α and β genes, of known restriction specificity, are introduced into the germline of mice by the microinjection of fertilized oocytes. The observation arising from the introduction of class I-restricted receptor genes has been that thymocytes expressing the transgene-encoded receptor are only clonally expanded and exported to the periphery if the appropriate MHC class I or class II molecule is expressed in the thymus. If the thymus of the transgenic mouse does not express the relevant MHC product, there appears to be a failure of positive selection such that cells expressing the transgene-encoded receptor do not appear in the peripheral immune system in significant numbers (Kisielow et al., 1988; Sha et al., 1988). The evidence for positive selection of the T-cell repertoire is summarized in Table 3.3.

Table 3.3 Evidence for positive selection

1. Bone marrow chimaeras	T-cells from {(A × B)F_1 into A} bone marrow chimaeras are restricted by thymic MHC type A
2. Thymus graft experiments	T-cells from (A × B)F_1 mice grafted with an A strain thymus are restricted by thymic MHC type A
3. T-cell receptor transgenic mice	The trangene-encoded T-cell receptors are only highly represented on peripheral T-cells if the MHC molecule that acts as the restriction element for the receptor is expressed in the thymus

Although the evidence for positive selection of the T-cell repertoire for self-MHC restriction is now very compelling, there are still some fundamental questions that remain unanswered. One such question is what role do self peptides play in the process of selection? As discussed earlier, it appears that most cell surface MHC molecules are occupied with peptides derived from the processing of self proteins. Thus it is likely that they contribute to the ligands that act as templates for the selection of receptors. Those that belong to the peptidic self school of thought would argue that peptides play the major role in positive selection, as they do (from this perspective) in peripheral T-cell recognition. However, this begs further questions. If the repertoire is selected on the basis of recognition of self peptides, why would that lead to self MHC-restricted recognition of foreign peptides, that are by definition different from the array of self peptides that were displayed in the thymus? Resolution of these complex issues may result from carefully designed transgenic experiments, leading to the expression of altered MHC molecules or aberrant peptides in the thymus. None the less, although many key questions regarding mechanisms remain unanswered, the original observations made almost two decades ago hold true. The T-cell repertoire is positively selected for the ability of its member T-cells to interact productively with host MHC products.

Negative selection

It has long been known that a high percentage of thymocytes, in the region of 98% (Scollay et al. 1980) dies within the thymus. One probable reason for thymocyte death is the failure to generate in-frame rearrangements of the TcR genes, so that no receptor dimer appears on the cell surface. It is clear, however, that a more active process is involved which reduces the risk of harmful autoreactions occurring. The dogma of clonal deletion as a mechanism of ensuring a safe T-cell repertoire, with minimal potential for autoreactivity, existed without any concrete experimental evidence for many years, after it was first proposed by Burnet in 1969. Once mAbs specific for individual TcR V segments became available it was possible to track the fate of receptors through the thymus. A spate of examples of clonal deletion followed the first report by Kappler et al. in 1987 of elimination of Vβ17a-expressing receptors in mice that expressed an H-2E MHC class II molecule. Several mouse MHC haplotypes carry a defect in either the H-2Ea or b gene so that no H-2E dimer is expressed, and in these strains they noted that approximately 10% of peripheral T-cells expressed the Vβ17a segment. The circle was completed when they also observed that Vβ17a-expressing T-cell hybridomas, derived from H-2E-negative mice, had a very high frequency of anti-H-2E alloreactivity. The sequel to these observations about H-2E reactivity and deletion of thymocytes expressing forbidden receptors, was a series of observations in mice that expressed the minor lymphocyte stimulating (Mls)-1^a allele. Mice that were Mls1^a-positive underwent intrathymic deletion of thymocytes bearing receptors containing Vβ6 (MacDonald et al., 1988) and Vβ8.1 segments (Kappler et al., 1988). As for the previous example, Vβ6- and Vβ8.1-expressing hybridomas isolated from Mls1^a-negative mice exhibited a very high frequency of anti-Mls1^a reactivity.

   Although these data provide clear instances of clonal deletion of thymocytes as a mechanism of self tolerance, it turns out that they are special cases and probably do not relate closely to the events that may lead to the deletion of self peptide-reactive T-cells. The reason for this is the observation that TcRs that include the Vβ17a segment do not see H-2E alone but co-recognize a cellular product which appears to be efficiently bound by most, if not all, H-2E types (Marrack and Kappler, 1988). Furthermore, the Vβ17a receptors are not classically MHC-restricted, and respond to most H-2E allelic types. Similarly, Mls1^a-reactive T-cells are dependent on the expression of a class II molecule by the stimulator cell, but there is little evidence of MHC restriction. The molecule responsible for the Mls1^a phenomenon has recently been defined as a product of the murine mammary tumour virus (Dyson et al., 1991; Marrack et al., 1991; Woodland et al., 1991). Indeed, additional retrovirus-derived deletion ligands have been identified in mice. It has yet to be established whether the same phenomena will exist in the selection of the human T-cell repertoire. It is a matter for conjecture as to whether the maintenance of the genes encoding these deletion ligands in the germline of the affected strains of mice is beneficial in some way. It could be that the deletions that occur render the repertoire of these mice safer in terms of autoreactive potential or in terms of unwanted toxic reactions to bacterial infections arising in later life.

These T-cell reactions mimic very closely those elicited by molecules that have been named superantigens such as the Staphylococcal enterotoxins. These superantigens do not behave according to the rules that apply to the majority of antigens in that they do not require to be processed, they are MHC-dependent but not MHC-restricted, and they probably do not bind within the peptide-binding groove of the MHC molecule. It has been proposed that they act as a bridge between a conserved region of an MHC molecule and particular Vβ segments (Janeway et al., 1989).

The best-defined example of clonal deletion as a mechanism of regulating what is almost certainly peptide-specific self-reactivity is the deletion, in the thymuses of transgenic male mice, of thymocytes bearing transgene-encoded receptors with specificity for the male antigen H-Y (Kisielow et al., 1988). In contrast, thymocytes expressing the same receptor in female mice of the same MHC type are not deleted and populate the peripheral lymphoid tissues. Assuming that this kind of clonal deletion is an important intra-thymic event, it should be possible to document further examples of the phenomenon, particularly when genes encoding polymorphic minor histocompatibility antigens are cloned and can be introduced into the thymus of a mouse that is otherwise negative for this antigen. However, it may be difficult to detect peptide-specific clonal elimination because the key regions of the TcR conferring peptide reactivity seem to be the clonally unique junctional sequences (Danska et al., 1990). More subtle approaches may be necessary to explore this issue in the future. The evidence for negative selection of the T-cell repertoire is summarized in Table 3.4.

In summary, it appears that the processes of positive and negative selection of developing thymocytes lead to the export of T-cells with intermediate affinity for host MHC molecules. This has been well articulated by Von Boehmer et al. (1989) who suggested that the thymus destroys the dangerous (autoreactive cells), ignores the useless (cells with very low affinity for thymic MHC products) and selects the useful

Table 3.4 Evidence for negative selection

1. Deletion of TcR Vβ families	Using monoclonal antibodies specific for individual Vβ families, intrathymic deletion of whole families was seen due to the expression of a molecule associated with the mouse MHC class II molecule H-2E (Vβ17a and Vβ11), or of the MMTV-encoded antigen Mls 1ᵃ (Vβ6 and Vβ8)
2. Deletion of TcR transgene-encoded receptors	T-cell receptor genes were introduced into the mouse germline as transgenes; it was noted that when the transgene-encoded receptors were specific for a thymically expressed self peptide, such as H-Y in male mice, thymocytes expressing the 'forbidden' receptor were deleted at the 'double positive' stage of thymic differentiation

(cells with intermediate affinity for thymic MHC molecules). Although the dogma is well in place, and well-supported, many of the molecular mechanisms that underlie these events are undefined. For example, how to account for the ability to impose the constraints of these two selective pressures on thymocytes using the same antigen receptor is one of the outstanding questions currently confronting T-cell immunologists.

Immune response gene effects

It was first noted in the late 1960s that genetically controlled differences existed in the magnitude of immune response following the immunization of inbred strains of animals. These phenomena were observed in guinea-pigs (Benacerraf et al., 1967) and in inbred mouse strains (Mitchell et al., 1972). The genes responsible for this variation were called immune response (Ir) genes. It was some years later that it became clear that Ir genes were, in most cases, one and the same as MHC genes. The definition of these effects in outbred human populations is much more difficult, but several HLA-linked examples have been described (Gotch et al., 1987; Sasazuki et al., 1989; Hill et al., 1991). This kind of HLA-linked immune response variation provides a very attractive mechanism to account for many HLA-linked diseases. Three major mechanisms to account for Ir gene effects have been characterized over the past ten years. These are discussed in turn below, and will be related to disease associations in a subsequent chapter.

Determinant selection

The concept from which this term derives is that individual MHC molecules select the determinants of an antigen that are displayed to T-cells restricted by that MHC molecule. The simplest way in which to visualize this selection operating is as the result of differing abilities of particular MHC types to bind and present individual antigenic peptides. In fact this concept was proposed long before any evidence was available in support of MHC:antigen association, and was a perceptive deduction from a series of functional data (Rosenthal and Sherach, 1973; Benacerraf, 1978). This topic was explored in extensive detail by Schwartz and colleagues using cytochrome c (cyt-c) as a model antigen. The results they obtained were referred to above, in the section on peptide/MHC association. They produced a series of cyt-c-specific mouse T-cell clones restricted by the murine MHC class II molecule H-2E^k, and defined their peptide specificity. The results are summarized in Table 3.5. Several clones were identified which exhibited limited degeneracy in that they were able to recognize both pigeon and moth cyt-c (residues 89–104), and they were able to use both H-2E^k or H-2E^b as a restriction element for recognition of the moth peptide. However, despite this degeneracy, no clones were seen which responded to pigeon cyt-c 89–104 together with H-2E^b (Heber-Katz et al., 1983). These data laid the blame for this failure of recognition very firmly at the feet of the H-2E^b molecule, and implied that it was unable to bind sufficient amounts of the pigeon peptide to trigger a response by these T-cells.

It became possible to test this theory directly when methods were developed to

Table 3.5   Recognition of cytochrome peptide 89–104 by H-2E-restricted mouse T-cell clones[a]

Peptide	Restriction element	
	H-2E^b	H-2E^k
Moth	+	+
Pigeon	–	+

[a] Data from Heber-Katz et al. (1983).

measure the physical association of peptides with MHC molecules. The first examples that were studied using equilibrium dialysis, as described above, demonstrated a clear correlation between the efficiency of MHC molecule/peptide association and known Ir gene effects for the peptide in question (Babbitt et al., 1985). In other words, an MHC molecule which bound the peptide under investigation efficiently was commonly used as a restriction element by T-cells specific for that peptide, and the converse was equally true. This analysis was applied to the interaction of the cyt-*c* peptide referred to above with H-2E^k and H-2E^b. The results were as predicted, in that pigeon cyt-*c* bound to H-2E^b ten times less well than to H-2E^k (Buus et al., 1987). This analysis was taken one stage further using recombinant H-2Eb genes, in which a hybrid β_1 domain-encoding exon was constructed such that the NH$_2$-terminal half of the domain was from H-2E^k (the haplotype that is able to present pigeon cyt-*c*) and the COOH-terminal half of the domain from H-2E^b (the non-functional haplotype for pigeon cyt-*c*). There is only a single amino-acid difference between these two alleles of H-2E in the NH$_2$-terminal half of the β_1 domain, the region which is predicted to encode the floor of the antigen-binding groove. This difference is at position 29, and would be predicted to influence peptide binding. Transfected cells expressing this hybrid b/k β_1 domain were fully able to present pigeon cyt-*c* to the T-cell clones described above (Ronchese et al., 1987), implying that the non-responder phenotype of H-2E^b for this peptide is explained by the inefficiency of peptide binding due to the influence of the substitution at position 29 in the floor of the groove. The concept of allele-specific patterns of peptide binding to MHC molecules has been well supported by the definition of naturally processed peptides, as discussed above. Little overlap was seen between the peptides eluted from the various class I molecules that have been studied. The data of Hill et al. (1992) is of particular interest in this regard, in that having observed a striking over-representation of the HLA class I type Bw53 in Zambia, an area where malaria is prevalent, he went on to show that the immunodominant peptide derived from a sporozoite protein bound preferentially to Bw53. This is an outstanding example of determinant selection having a clear-cut effect on immune protection against an environmental agent.

However, in contrast to examples such as pigeon cyt-*c* and H-2E, there are well-documented instances in which there is no correlation between the ability of a peptide to associate with an MHC product and its recognition with that MHC molecule. This is reviewed by Buus et al. (1987). Clearly other mechanisms underlie some Ir gene effects, as discussed below.

Holes in the T-cell repertoire

Bearing in mind the extensive deletion of differentiating thymocytes with self-reactive specificities, it might be predicted that gaps or holes may be created in the exported repertoire of T-cells, that manifest as a failure to recognize some extrinsic antigens. It would be predicted that the dominant genetic factor leading to the presence of such gaps would be the inheritance of individual MHC alleles. Long before current concepts of the tri-molecular complex of TcR, MHC molecule and peptide had evolved, Mullbacher (1981) described an Ir gene effect that appeared to be best accounted for by the existence of a hole in the repertoire. They observed that in $(b \times s)$ F_1 mice the cytotoxic T-cell response to the male-specific minor transplantation antigen H-Y was almost entirely restricted by H-2^s class I molecules, and the H-2^b-restricted response to H-Y was barely detectable. In contrast, homozygous H-2^b mice were able to generate strong H-Y-specific responses. In other words the presence of H-2^s-encoded MHC molecules in some way caused a marked reduction in the H-2^b-restricted response to H-Y. The clue to the mechanism underlying this phenomenon was provided by studying H-2^b-restricted H-Y-specific T-cells raised from homozygous H-2^b mice. T-cells with this specificity turned out to cross-react strongly on allogeneic H-2^s cells in the absence of the male-specific antigen. These data suggest that H-2^s class I molecules, as expressed in the thymus, mimic H-2^b + H-Y, and that as a consequence T-cells with the potential for recognizing H-2^b + H-Y are deleted in the thymus of $(b \times s)$ F_1 mice, because of autoreactivity against H-2^s class I molecules. These were very elegant experiments, however, limited additional examples exist in support of holes in the repertoire as a mechanism of Ir gene effects. This probably reflects the fact that designing suitable experiments is far from easy, rather than that this is an unimportant mechanism.

T-cell-mediated suppression

The third major mechanism proposed to account for MHC-linked Ir gene effects invokes active regulation of potentially reactive cells by a population of cells whose specialist function is to suppress antigen reactivity. The idea that cells existed whose function it is to suppress an immune response was first proposed by Gershon in 1974. Such cells would be the opposite of helper T-cells and would act to prevent unwanted immunity, and perhaps serve to make immune responses self-limiting. A huge literature has accumulated on the subject of suppressor cells over the past 20 years, and many immunologists have travelled up a number of blind alleys. None the less, there are some very clear-cut and reproducible examples of genetically determined non-responsiveness that appears to result from the action of suppressor cells with a T-cell phenotype (Ts).

In response to the antigen hen egg lysozyme (HEL), mice of the H-2^b haplotype are non-responders, in contrast to H-2^k animals that make a strong response. In exploring this immune response variation, Sercasz and colleagues made two important observations. The first was that removal of the NH$_2$- and COOH-terminal fragments of the HEL molecule by enzymatic cleavage, converted H-2^b mice into responders (Adorini et al., 1979). This result gave rise to the idea that antigens carried distinct suppressor (as well as helper) determinants. It also made clear that HEL peptides were capable of binding to H-2^b MHC products, and thus that determinant selection could not be the sole explanation for this Ir gene effect. Similarly, it made clear that T-cells are present in the repertoire of H-2^b mice that are able to recognize HEL peptides efficiently. The second observation arose from mixing experiments, in which the T-cells from an H-2^b mouse that had been primed with intact HEL were mixed with cells from a second mouse that had been immunized with the truncated HEL molecule. The consistent finding was that the T-cells from the first mouse completely suppressed the response of the second mouse, implying that the non-responsiveness of H-2^b mice was due, at least in part, to the effect of suppressor cells.

Some of the clearest evidence in support of the existence of specialized Ts has been derived from experimental models of organ transplantation. Several groups have reported the observation that animals carrying an established kidney or heart allograft possess Ts, which can be adoptively transferred to a naive syngeneic recipient and provide protection for a freshly transplanted graft from the same strain as the graft residing in the Ts donor (Marquet et al., 1981; Horsburgh et al., 1983). These cells are specific for the donor strain, and have been variously reported to be of the CD4 and of the CD8 phenotype.

Although these examples provide strong support for the existence of suppressor T-cells, many questions about Ts remain unresolved. The major uncertainty is about their specificity. Two major models have been proposed, the first is that they are antigen-specific, and interact with the same APC as the Th or Tc which they suppress. The second is that they have specificity for the antigen receptor on the target cell which they suppress. This second model has been extensively studied by Engelman (for review, see Mohagheghpour et al., 1986) and discussed recently by Batchelor and colleagues (1989). Until stable clones of Ts are obtained which can be characterized in detail, this issue will remain unresolved. The minimalist view of suppressor phenomena is that they are mediated passively by antigen-specific T-cells that have been rendered tolerant, but retain cell-surface receptor expression. It has been argued by Waldmann and colleagues (Waldmann et al., 1992) that such cells have the capacity to compete for the available antigen:MHC molecule complexes, and thus deprive potentially reactive T-cells from obtaining sufficient productive interactions in order to be activated. The attraction of this hypothesis is that it imposes no requirement for a separate population of T-cells with distinct specificities or effector functions.

A related perspective is that suppressor cells are simply a population of T-cells with entirely overlapping specificity with conventional helper cells, but that the distinctive feature of suppressor cells is that they secrete a cocktail of lymphokines that is inhibitory to neighbouring T-cells. This suggestion has received support from the recent elucidation of two subpopulations of CD4$^+$ T-cells that are characterized by the secretion of different cocktails of cytokines. One subpopulation, referred to as the T helper 1 (Th1) subset, secretes predominantly IL-2 and γ-interferon (γ-IFN), the other subpopulation secretes predominantly IL-4 and IL-10 and is referred to as the Th2 subset. The relevance of these findings to the phenomena of suppression is that the cytokines secreted by these two subpopulations of cells regulate the activities of the other subpopulation. For example, IL-4 and IL-10 inhibit the secretion of IL-2, and γ-IFN inhibits the secretion of IL-4. These observations, and their potential in vivo relevance is reviewed by Fowell and colleagues (1991).

Conclusion

It has become clear during the past two decades that MHC molecules play a central role in the generation of specific immune responses. This is the consequence of their functions of selecting the mature T-cell repertoire during thymic differentiation, and of binding and displaying peptides derived from intact proteins for T-cell recognition. The extensive intra-allelic polymorphism that these molecules exhibit is reflected in immune response gene variation. The mechanisms underlying this variation are increasingly well understood, and are likely to be responsible for at least some of the known HLA and disease associations. This will be discussed in more detail in Chapter 5.

References

Adorini, L., Harvey, M. A., Miller, A. et al. (1979). Fine specificity of regulatory cells – II suppressor and helper T cells are induced by different regions of hen egg-white lysozyme in a genetically nonresponder mouse strain. *J.Exp.Med.* **150**: 293–306.

Ajitkumar, P., Geier, S.S., Kesari, K.V. et al. (1988). Evidence that multiple residues on both the α-helices of the class I MHC molecule are simultaneously recognized by the T cell receptor. *Cell* **54**: 47–56.

Allen, P., Matsueda, G., Evans, R. et al. (1987). Identification of the T-cell and Ia contact residues of a T-cell antigenic epitope. *Nature* **327**: 713–715.

Babbit, B.P., Allen, P.M., Matsueda, G. et al. (1985). Binding of immunogenic peptides to Ia histocompatibility molecules. *Nature* **317**: 359–361.

Bakke, O. and Dobberstein, B. (1990). MHC class II-associated invariant chain contains a sorting signal for endosomal compartments. *Cell* **63**: 707–716.

Barber, L.D., Bal, V., Lamb, J.R. et al. (1991). Contribution of T-cell receptor-contacting and peptide-binding residues of the class II molecule HLA-DR4 Dw10 to serologic and antigen-specific T-cell recognition. *Hum. Immunol.* **32**: 110–118.

Batchelor, J.R., Lombardi, G. and Lechler, R.I. (1989). Speculations on the specificity of suppression. *Immunol. Today* **10**: 37–40.

Benacerraf, B. (1978). A hypothesis to relate the specificity of T lymphocytes and the activity of I region-specific Ir genes in macrophages and B lymphocytes. *J. Immunol.* **120**: 1809–1812.

Benacerraf, B., Green, I. and Paul, W.E. (1967). The immune response of guinea pigs to hapten-poly-L-lysine conjugates as an example of the genetic control of the recognition of antigenicity. *Cold Spring Harb. Symp. Quant. Biol.* **32**: 569–576.

Bevan, M.J. (1977). In a radiation chimaera host H-2 antigens determine immune responsiveness of donor cytotoxic cells. *Nature* **269**: 417–418.

Bikoff, E., Huang, L.-Y., Episkopou, V. et al. (1993). Defective major histocompatibility complex class II assembly, transport, peptide acquisition, and CD4+T cell selection in mice lacking invariant chain expression. *J.Exp.Med.* **177**: 1699–1712.

Bjorkman, P.J., Saper, M.A., Samraoui, N. et al. (1987). Structure of the human class I histocompatibility antigen, HLA-A2. *Nature* **329**: 506–512.

Brenner, M.B., McLean, J. Dialynas, D.P. et al. (1986). Identification of a putative second T-cell receptor. *Nature* **322**: 145–149.

Brent, L. and Opara, S.C. (1979). Specific unresponsiveness to skin allografts in mice. V. Synergy between donor tissue extract, procarbazine hydrochloride and antilymphocyte serum in creating a long lasting unresponsiveness mediated by suppressor T cells. *Transplantation* **27**: 120–126.

Brown, J.H., Jardetzky, T., Saper, M.A. et al. (1988). A hypothetical model of the foreign antigen binding site of class II histocompatibility molecules. *Nature* **332**: 845–850.

Burnet, M. (1969). *Cellular Immunology.* Melbourne University Press, Carlton.

Buus, S., Sette, A., Colon, S.M. et al. (1987). The relation between major histocompatibility complex (MHC) restriction and the capacity of Ia to bind immunogenic peptides. *Science* **235**: 1353–1357.

Cammarota, G., Scheirle, A., Takacs, B. et al. (1992). Identification of a CD4 binding site on the β_2 domain of HLA-DR molecules. *Nature* **356**: 799–801.

Chen, B.P., Madrigal, A. and Parham, P. (1990). Cytotoxic T cell recognition of an endogenous class I HLA peptide presented by a class II HLA molecule. *J. Exp. Med.* **172**: 779–788.

Chicz, R.M., Urban, R.G., Lane, W.S. et al. (1992). Predominant naturally processed peptides bound to HLA-DR1 are derived from MHC-related molecules and are heterogenous in size. *Nature* **358**: 764–768.

Chien, Y., Becker, D.M., Lindsten, T. et al. (1984). A third type of murine T-cell receptor gene. *Nature* **312**: 31–35.

Claverie, J.M. and Kourilsky, P. (1986). The peptidic self model: a hypothesis on the molecular nature of the immunological self. *Ann. Inst. Pasteur Immunol.* **137D**: 3–21.

Danska, J.S., Livingston, A.M., Paragas, V. et al. (1990). The presumptive CDR3 regions of both T cell receptor α and β chains determine T cell specificity for myoglobin peptides. *J. Exp. Med.* **172**: 27–33.

Davis, M.M. and Bjorkman, P.J. (1988). T cell receptor genes and T cell recognition. *Nature* **334**: 395–402.

DeLisi, C. and Berzofsky, J. (1985). T-cell antigenic sites tend to be amphipathic structures. *Proc. Natl Acad. Sci. USA* **82**: 7048–7052.

Deverson, E.V., Gow, I.R., Coadwell, W.J. et al. (1990). MHC Class II region encoding proteins related to the multidrug resistance family of transmembrane transporters. *Nature* **348**: 738–741.

Dialynas, D.P., Wilde, D., Marrack, P. et al. (1983). Characterization of the murine antigenic determinant L3T4a, recognised by monoclonal antibody GK1.5: Expression of L3T4a by functional T cell clones appears to correlate primarily with class II MHC antigen reactivity. *Immunol. Rev.* **74**: 29–56.

Doyle, C. and Strominger, J.L. (1987). Interaction between CD4 and class II MHC molecules mediates cell adhesion. *Nature* **330**: 256–259.

Dyson, P.J., Knight, A.M., Fairchild, S. et al. (1991). Genes encoding ligands for deletion of Vβ11 T cells cosegregate with mammary tumour virus genomes. *Nature* **349**: 531–532.

Eichmann, K., Jonsson, J.-I., Falk, I. et al. (1987). Effective activation of resting mouse T lymphocytes by cross-lining submitogenic concentrations of the T cell antigen receptor with either Lyt-2 or L3T4. *Eur. J. Immunol.* **17**: 643–650.

Falk, K., Rotzschke, O. and Rammensee, H.G. (1990). Cellular peptide composition governed by major histocompatibility complex class I molecules. *Nature* **348**: 248–251.

Fink, P. and Bevan, M. (1978). H-2 antigens of the thymus determine lymphocyte specificity. *J. Exp. Med.* **148**: 766–778.

Fink, P., Matis, L., McEllingot, L. et al. (1986). Correlations between T-cell specificity and the structure of the antigen receptor. *Nature* **321**: 219–226.

Fowell, D., McKnight, A., Powrie, F. et al. (1991). Subsets of CD4$^+$ T cells and their roles in the induction and prevention of autoimmunity. *Immunol. Rev.* **123**: 37–64.

Frankel, W.N., Rudy, C., Coffin, J.M. et al. (1991). Linkage of MIs genes to endogenous mammary tumour viruses of inbred mice. *Nature* **349**: 526–527.

Garrett, T.P.J., Saper, M.A., Bjorkman, P.J. et al. (1989). Specificity pockets for the side chains of peptide antigens in HLA-Aw68. *Nature* **342**: 692–696.

Germain, R. (1986). The ins and outs of antigen processing and presentation. *Nature* **322**: 687–689.

Germain, R.N. and Rinker Jr., A.G. (1993). Peptide binding inhibits protein aggregation of invariant-chain free class II dimers and promotes surface expression of occupied molecules. *Nature* **363**: 725–728.

Gershon, R. (1974). T-cell control of antibody production. *Contemp. Top. Immunobiol.* **3**: 1–40.

Gotch, F.M., Rothbard, J., Howland, K. et al. (1987). Cytotoxic T lymphocytes recognize a fragment of influenza virus matrix protein in association with HLA-A2. *Nature* **326**: 881–885.

Glynne, R., Powis, S.H. et al. (1991). A proteasome-related gene between the two ABC transporter loci in the class II region of the human MHC. *Nature* **353**: 357–360.

Gorer, P.A. (1938). The antigenic basis of tumour transplantation. *J. Path. Bact.* **47**: 231–252.

Grey, H.M., Colon, S.M. and Chestnut, R.W. (1982). Requirements for the processing of antigen by antigen-presenting B cells. II. Biochemical comparison of the fate of antigen in B cell tumours and macrophages. *J. Immunol.* **129**: 2389–2395.

Hammer, J., Takacs, B. and Sinigaglia, F. (1992). Identification of a motif for HLA-DR1 binding peptides using M13 display libraries. J. Exp. Med. **176**: 1007–1013.

Heber-Katz, E., Hansburg, D. and Schwartz, R.H. (1983). The Ia molecule of the antigen-presenting cell plays a critical role in immune response gene regulation of T cell activation. *J. Mol. Cell Immunol.* **1**: 3–14.

Hedrick, S.M., Nielsen, E.A., Kavaler, J. et al. (1984). Sequence relationships between putative T-cell receptor polypeptides and immunoglobulins. *Nature* **308**: 153–158.

Hill, A.V.S., Allsopp, C.E.M., Kwiatkowski, D. et al. (1991). Common West African HLA antigens are associated with protection from severe malaria. *Nature* **352**: 565–600.

Hill, A.V.S., Elvin, J., Willis, A.C. et al. (1992). Molecular analysis of the association of HLA-B53 and resistance to severe malaria. *Nature* **360**: 434–439.

Horsburgh, T., Wood, P.J. and Brent, L. (1983). In vivo induction of specific suppressor lymphocytes to histocompatibility antigen. *Trans. Proc.* **13**: 637–639.

Hunt, D.F., Henderson, R.A., Shabanowitz, J. et al. (1992). Characterization of peptides bound to the Class I MHC molecule HLA-A2.1 by Mass spectrometry. *Science* **255**: 1261–1263.

Jacobson, S., Sekaly, R.P., Jacobson, C.L. et al. (1989). HLA class II-restricted presentation of cytoplasmic measles virus antigens to cytotoxic T cells. *J. Virol.* **63**: 1756–1762.

Janeway, C.A., Yagi, J., Conrad, P.J. et al. (1989). T-cell responses to Mls and to bacterial proteins that mimic its behavior. *Immunol. Rev.* **107**: 61–88.

Jardetzky, T.S., Lane, W.S., Robinson, R.A. et al. (1991). Identification of self peptides bound to purified HLA-B27. *Nature* **353**: 326–328.

Kappler, J.W., Roehm, N. and Marrack, P. (1987). T cell tolerance by clonal elimination in the thymus. *Cell* **49**: 273–280.

Kappler, J.W., Skidmore, B., White, J. et al. (1981). Antigen-inducible, H-2-restricted, interleukin-2-producing T cell hybridomas. Lack of independent antigen and H-2 recognition. *J. Exp. Med.* **153**: 1198–1214.

Kappler, J.W., Staerz, U., White, J. et al. (1988). Self tolerance eliminates T cell specific for MLs-modified products of the major histocompatibility complex. *Nature* **332**: 35–40.

Kisielow, P., Sia Teh, H., Bluthmann, H. et al. (1988). Positive selection of antigen-specific T cells in thymus by restricting MHC molecules. *Nature* **335**: 730–733.

König, R., Huang, L.Y. and Germain, R.N. (1992). MHC class II interaction with CD4 mediated by a region analogous to the MHC class I binding site for CD8. *Nature* **356**: 796–798.

Kupfer, A., Singer, S.J., Janeway, C.A. et al. (1987). Co-clustering of CD4 (L3T4) molecule with the T-cell receptor is induced by specific direct interaction of helper T cells and antigen-presenting cells. *Proc. Natl Acad. Sci. USA* **84**: 5888–5892.

Lee, P., Matsueda, G.R. and Allen, P.M. (1988). T-cell recognition of fibrinogen. A determinant of the α-chain does not require processing. *J. Immunol.* **140**: 1063–1068.

Ljunggren, H-G., Stam, N., Ohlen, C. et al. (1990). Empty MHC class I molecules come out in the cold. *Nature* **346**: 476–480.

Lo, D. and Sprent, J. (1986). Identity of cells that imprint H-2-restricted T-cell specificity in the thymus. *Nature* **319**: 672–675.

Lombardi, G., Barber, L., Aichinger, G. et al. (1991). Structural analysis of anti-DR1 allorecognition by using DR1/H-2E^k hybrid molecules. *J. Immunol.* **147**: 2034–2040.

MacDonald, H.R., Schneider, R., Lees, R.K. et al. (1988). T-cell receptor Vβ use predicts reactivity and tolerance to Mls^a-encoded antigens. *Nature* **332**: 40–45.

Madden, D.R., Gorga, J.C., Strominger, J.L. et al. (1991). The structure of HLA-B27 reveals nonamer self-peptides bound in an extended conformation. *Nature* **353**: 321–325.

Malnati, M., Marti, M., LaVaute, T. et al. (1992). Processing pathways for presentation of cytosolic antigen to MHC class II-restricted T cells. *Nature* **357**: 702–704.

Marquet, R.L. and Heyskek, G.A. (1981). Induction of suppressor cells by donor-specific blood transfusions and heart transplantation in rats. *Transplantation* **31**: 271–274.

Marrack, P. and Kappler, J.W. (1988). T cells can distinguish between allogeneic major histocompatibility complex products on different cell types. *Nature* **332**: 840–843.

Marrack, P., Kushnir, E., Born, W. et al. (1988). The development of helper T cell precursors in mouse thymus. *J. Immunol.* **140**: 2508–2514.

Marrack, P., Kushnir, E. and Kappler, J.A. (1991). Maternally inherited superantigen encoded by a mammary tumour virus. *Nature* **349**: 524–525.

Mitchell, G.F., Grumet, F.C. and McDevitt, H.O. (1972). Genetic Control of the Immune Response: The effect of thymectomy on the primary and secondary antibody response of mice to poly-l (Tyr,Glu)-poly-d, l-Ala--poly-l-Lys. *J. Exp. Med.* **135**: 126–135.

Mohagheghpour, N., Damle, N.K. and Takada, S.J. et al. (1986). Generation of antigen receptor-specific suppressor T cell clones in man. *J. Exp. Med.* **164**: 950–955.

Monaco, J.J., Cho, S. and Attaya, M. (1990). Transport protein genes in the murine MHN: possible implications for antigen processing. *Science* **250**: 1723–1726.

Moore, M.W., Carbone, F.R. and Bevan, M.J. (1988). Introduction of soluble protein into the class I pathway of antigen processing and presentation. *Cell* **54**: 777–785.

Moreno, J., Vignali, D.A.A., Nadimi, F. et al. (1991). Processing of an endogenous protein can generate MHC class II-restricted T cell determinants distinct from those derived from exogenous antigen. *J. Immunol.* **147**: 3306–3313.

Morrison, L.A., Lukacher, A.E., Braciale, V.L. et al. (1986). Differences in antigen presentation to MHC class I- and class II-restricted influenza virus-specific cytolytic T lymphocyte clones. *J. Exp. Med.* **163**: 903–921.

Mullbacher, A., Sheena, J.H., Fierz, W. et al. (1981). Specific haplotype preference in congenic F1 hybrid mice in the cytotoxic T cell response to the male specific antigen H-Y. *J. Immun.* 127(2): 686–689.

Patten, P., Yokota, T., Rothbard, J. et al. (1984). Structure, expression and divergence of T-cell receptor β-chain variable regions. *Nature* 312: 40–46.

Paul, W.E., Shevach, E.M., Pickeral, S. et al. (1977). Independent populations of primed F1 guinea pig: T lymphocytes respond to antigen-pulsed parental peritoneal exudate cells. *J. Exp. Med.* 145: 618–629.

Peterson, M. and Miller, J. (1990). Invariant chain influences the immunological recognition of MHC class II molecules. *Nature* 345: 172–174.

Potter, T.A., Rajan, T.V., Dick, R.F. et al. (1989). Substitution at residue 227 of H-2 class I molecules abrogates recognition by CD8-dependent, but not CD8-independent, cytotoxic lymphocytes. *Nature* 337: 73–75.

Roche, P.A. and Cresswell, P. (1990). Invariant chain association with HLA-DR molecules inhibits immunogenic peptide binding. *Nature* 345: 615–618.

Ronchese, F., Schwartz, R.H. and Germain, R.N. (1987). Functionally distinct subsites on a class II major histocompatibility complex molecule. *Nature* 329: 254–256.

Rosenthal, H.S. and Shevach, E.M. (1973). Function of macrophages in antigen recognition by guinea pig T lymphocytes I. Requirement for histocompatible macrophages and lymphocytes. *J. Exp. Med.* 138: 1194–1212.

Rotzke, O. and Falk, K. (1991). Naturally occurring peptide antigens derived from the MHC class I-restricted processing pathway. *Immunol. Today* 12: 447–455.

Rudensky, A.Y., Preston-Hurlburt, P. and Hong, S.C. (1991). Sequence analysis of peptides bound to MHC class II molecules. *Nature* 353: 622–627.

Saito, H., Kranz, D.M., Takagaki, Y. et al. (1984). A third rearranged and expressed gene in a clone of cytotoxic T lymphocytes. *Nature* 312: 36–40.

Salter, R.D., Benjamin, R.J., Wesley, P.K. et al. (1990). A binding site for the T-cell co-receptor CD8 on the α3 domain of HLA-A2. *Nature* 345: 41–46.

Samelson, L.E., Germain, R.N. and Schwartz, R.H. (1983). Monoclonal antibodies against the antigen receptor on a cloned T-cell hybrid. *Proc. Natl Acad. Sci. USA* 80: 6972–6976.

Sasazuki, T., Kikuchi, I., Hirayama, K. et al. (1989). HLA-linked immune suppression in humans. *Immunology* 2: 21–24.

Scollay, R.G., Butcher, E.C. and Weissman, I.L. (1980). Thymus cell migration. Quantitative aspects of cellular traffic from the thymus to the periphery in mice. *Eur. J. Immunol.* 10: 210–218.

Sha, W.C., Nelson, C.A., Newberry, R.D. et al. (1988). Selective expression of an antigen receptor on CD8-bearing T lymphocytes in transgenic mice. *Nature* 335: 271–274.

Shimonkevitz, R., Colon, S., Kappler, J.W. et al. (1984). Antigen recognition by H-2 restricted T cells II. A tryptic ovalbumin peptide that substitutes for processed antigen. *J. Immunol.* 133: 2067–2074.

Spies, T., Bresnahan, M., Bahram, S. et al. (1990). A gene in the human major histocompatibility complex class II region controlling the class I antigen presentation pathway. *Nature* 348: 744–747.

Stockinger, B., Pessara, U., Lin, R.H. et al. (1989). A role of Ia-associated invariant chains in antigen processing and presentation. *Cell* 56: 683–689.

Swain, S.L. (1981). Significance of Lyt phenotypes: Lyt-2 antibodies block activities of T-cells that recognize class I major histocompatibility complex antigens regardless of their function. *Proc. Natl Acad. Sci. USA* 78: 7101–7105.

Teyton, L., O'Sullivan, D., Dickson, P.W. et al. (1990). Invariant chain distinguishes between the exogenous and endogenous antigen presentation pathways. *Nature* 348: 39–45.

Thomas, D.B., Hodgson, J., Riska, P.F. et al. (1990). The role of the endoplasmatic reticulum in antigen processing. N-glycosylation of influenza hemagglutinin abrogates CD4$^+$ cytotoxic T cell recognition of endogenously processed antigen. *J. Immunol.* 144: 2789–2794.

Townsend, A.R.M., Gotch, F.M. and Davey, J. (1985). Cytotoxic T cells recognize fragments of influenza nucleoprotein *Cell* 42: 457.

Townsend, A.R.M., Bastin, J., Gould, K. et al. (1986). Cytotoxic T lymphocytes recognise influenza haemagglutinin that lacks a signal sequence. *Nature* 324: 575–577.

Townsend, A., Ohlen, C., Bastin, J. et al. (1989). Association of class I major histocompatibility heavy and light chains induced by viral peptides. *Nature* 340: 443–448.

Trowsdale, J., Hanson, I., Mockridge, I. et al. (1990). Sequences encoded in the class II region of the MHC related to the 'ABC' superfamily of transporters. *Nature* 348: 741–743.

Veillette, A., Bookman, M.A., Horak, E.M. et al. (1988). The CD4 and CD8 T cell surface antigens are associated with the internal membrane tyrosine-protein kinase p56^{lck}. *Cell* 55: 301–308.

Viville, S., Neefjes, J., Lotteau, V. et al. (1993). Mice lacking the MHC Class II-Associated Invariant Chain. *Cell* **72**: 635–648.

Von Boehmer, H., Teh, H.S. and Kisielow, P. (1989). The thymus selects the useful, neglects the useless and destroys the harmful. *Immunol. Today* **10**: 57–61.

Waldmann, H., Qin, S. and Cobbold, S. (1992). Monoclonal antibodies as agents to reinduce tolerance in autoimmunity. *J. Autoimmunity* **5**: 93–102.

Woodland, D.L., Happ, M.P., Gollob, K.J. et al. (1991). An endogenous retrovirus mediating deletion of αβ T cells. *Nature* **349**: 529–530.

Yanagi, Y.Y., Yoshikai, Y., Leggett, K. et al. (1984). A human T cell-specific cDNA clone encodes a protein having extensive homology to immunoglobulin chains. *Nature* **308**: 145–149.

Ziegler, K. and Unanue, E.R. (1981). Identification of a macrophage antigen-processing event required for I-region restricted antigen presentation to T lymphocytes. *J. Immunol.* **127**: 1869–1875.

Zinkernagel, R.M. and Doherty, P.C. (1975). H-2 Compatibility requirement for T-cell-mediated lysis of target cells infected with lymphocytic choriomeningitis virus. *J. Exp. Med.* **141**: 1427–1436.

Zinkernagel, R.M., Callahan, G.N., Althage, A. et al. (1978). On the thymus in the differentiation of 'H-2 self-recognition' by T cells: evidence for dual recognition? *J. Exp. Med.* **147**: 882–896.

CHAPTER 4

Expression of class I and class II MHC molecules: influence of the induction of MHC class II expression on tolerance and autoimmunity

Robert Lechler
Department of Immunology
Royal Postgraduate Medical School
London, UK

The distribution of the two classes of MHC molecule bears a very logical relationship with the functions of these products in immune responses, as discussed in Chapter 2. Class I molecules are expressed on almost all nucleated cells, with the exception of central nervous system neurones, corneal endothelium, exocrine cells of the pancreas, and placental trophoblast cells in some species. Constitutive expression of class II molecules is restricted to a limited number of cell types, mainly on specialized antigen-presenting cells of bone marrow origin, and on thymic cortical epithelial cells to enable positive selection of differentiating thymocytes. As discussed in Chapter 3, class I-restricted presentation of antigen requires that the antigen is synthesized inside the presenting cell. Given that the large majority of cytotoxic T-cells are class I-restricted, this means that any virus-infected cell, with a small number of exceptions, can be lysed by Tc. In contrast, most peptides that are presented with MHC class II products appear to be derived from antigens that are internalized by the presenting cell, or that are membrane-bound molecules. Most T-cells of the helper phenotype are class II-restricted, so that class II-expressing cells which have ingested virus or viral antigens, but are not actually infected, will stimulate T-cell help through class II-restricted presentation, but will avoid lysis by class I-restricted Tc.

The genetic basis of MHC gene regulation, and tissue specificity is a large and complex topic, which there is not space to cover here. The current state of knowledge of this subject was discussed in Chapter 1, and is well reviewed by David-Watine et al. (1990).

HLA and Disease
ISBN 0–12–440320–4

Inductive stimuli for MHC class II expression

Although constitutive expression of MHC class II molecules is limited to a small number of cell lineages, class II molecule expression can be induced on a wide variety of cell types. These include endothelial cells, epithelial cells at multiple sites including the lactating breast, fibroblasts, keratinocytes, astrocytes, and human T-cells (reviewed in Klareskog and Forsum, 1986). It is interesting, though not explained, that the induction of class II expression on activated T-cells is widely observed in man, but seems not to occur at all in the mouse. The immunological significance of class II induction at all these different sites will be discussed below. Before doing so, there are two other aspects of MHC class II expression that contribute to individual variation, and may vary under the stress of inductive stimuli, but are often overlooked.

Regulation of αβ chain assembly and cell surface expression

As described in Chapter 1, class II molecules are heterodimers composed of an α and a β chain which are non-covalently associated at the cell surface. The rules that govern the process of αβ chain assembly and cell surface expression have emerged during the past few years, largely as the result of an extensive series of gene transfection experiments. It has become clear that αβ dimers of the mouse H-2A and the human HLA-DQ class II loci that are encoded in *cis*, on the same haplotype, are most efficiently expressed. However, *trans* pairs composed of haplotype-mismatched α and β chains, can also be expressed at the cell surface with a range of efficiencies dictated by the particular alleles involved. For example, the allelically mismatched H-2A pairs $A\alpha^b A\beta^k$ and $A\alpha^k A\beta^b$ are expressed at the surface of cells transfected with the appropriate genes with comparable efficiency to the allelically matched pairs $A\alpha^b A\beta^b$ and $A\alpha^k A\beta^k$. In contrast it seems to be impossible to achieve cell surface expression of the haplotype-mismatched pair $A\alpha^k A\beta^d$ (Braunstein and Germain, 1987). Direct evidence in support of the expression of haplotype-mismatched αβ dimers was described by Beck et al. (1982) some years before these transfection experiments, who defined T-cell clones from $(b \times k)F_1$ mice which were restricted by the F_1-specific molecules, $A\alpha^b A\beta^k$ or $A\alpha^k A\beta^b$. Similar rules have been shown to apply to the expression of αβ dimers of HLA-DQ (Kwok et al., 1988). These observations are illustrated diagramatically in Figure 4.1. Furthermore, following the transfection of the locus- (isotype-)mismatched pair of murine class II genes H-2Ea and H-2Ab^d, cell surface expression was detected (Quill et al., 1985). Of the three alleles of Aβ that were tested in these experiments, Aβ^d was the only one that appeared able to associate with the invariant Eα chain, demonstrating that the assembly and expression of isotype-mismatched αβ dimers is also under allelic control. The expression of a mismatched dimer, such as $E\alpha A\beta^d$, in a transfected cell which is not expressing the genes encoding the isotype-matched α and β chains, clearly does not mean that the same molecule would be expressed in a normal cell in which isotype-matched αβ pairs are likely to compete effectively for the assembly of such a mismatched molecule. It was of considerable interest that the human equivalent molecule to $E\alpha A\beta^d$, namely DRαDQβ, was detected at the surface of a transformed B-cell line by immunoprecipitation (Lotteau et al., 1987). Pursuing the issue of isotype-mismatched αβ chain

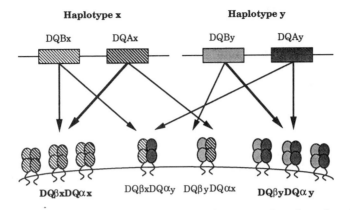

Figure 4.1 The four possible DQ heterodimers that can be expressed at the cell surface of a DQ heterozygous class II-positive cell are represented. As indicated by the bold arrows, and the larger number of class II dimers, *cis* pairing is favoured over *trans* pairing. As discussed in the text, the extent of haplotype-mismatched assembly and expression is determined by the class II alleles carried by the two haplotypes.

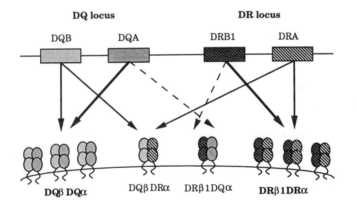

Figure 4.2 The possible isotype-mismatched class II heterodimers that can arise from the α and β chains encoded at the DR and DQ loci are shown. As discussed in the text, evidence exists for the cell surface expression of DRβDQα, however, no evidence exists to suggest that the reciprocal dimer can be expressed. As for the expression of haplotype-mismatched dimers, the assembly and expression of isotype-mismatched dimers appears to be influenced by allelic polymorphism in the class II molecules.

assembly and expression, Sant and Germain generated three gene transfectants, containing Ea and Ab^d genes together with either the Eb^d or the Aa^d gene (Sant and Germain, 1989). They then compared the levels of cell surface expression of the mixed isotype molecule, EαAβ^d, with the levels of the isotype-matched αβ dimers, and correlated these with the levels of messenger RNA. They concluded from these studies that there was at least a ten-fold higher efficiency of isotype matched versus mismatched dimer formation. The formation of isotype-mismatched dimers is illustrated in Figure 4.2.

The implication of these relative efficiencies of αβ dimer formation is that isotype-mismatched and unfavourable haplotype-mismatched αβ dimers will only be expressed at very low levels on the surface of normal cells. Higher levels may arise under circumstances in which there is an imbalance in the molar ratio of α and β chains synthesized inside a cell (Lechler, 1988). It could be envisaged that this would occur under the stress of an inductive stimulus, such as may arise at the site of an inflammatory response. This kind of non-stoichiometry of α and β chains has been artificially created in a human B cell by transfecting an anti-sense construct of the DRB gene into a human B cell line. The consequent excess of DRα polypeptides led to the cell surface expression of a DRαDQβ molecule (Lotteau et al., 1989).

The important question is whether particular αβ dimers are expressed at levels sufficient to act as restriction elements for T-cell recognition. This question was clearly answered by the detection of T-cells from H-2^d mice, immunized with the experimental antigen sperm-whale myoglobin, that were restricted by the isotype-mismatched molecule Aβ^{d}Eα. All the T-cells with specificity for one peptide fragment of this antigen were restricted by this class II molecule, and did not respond to peptide presented by native H-2A^d or H-2E^d (Ruberti et al., 1991). Although this may prove to be a rare event, and may be explained by the binding of this myoglobin peptide to the mismatched molecule with particularly high affinity, these observations provide direct evidence that class II molecules such as the Aβ^{d}Eα dimer can be expressed at sufficient levels to act as restriction elements for T-cells.

The potential relevance of all this to autoimmunity and disease pathogenesis lies in the possibility that a mismatched αβ MHC class II molecule may be over-expressed during the course of an immune response, at levels to which the T-cell repertoire is not tolerant, because such a molecule was only expressed at low levels in the thymus during T-cell ontogeny. Presentation of an autoantigen by such a molecule could lead to the development of an autoimmune reaction.

Heterogeneity in cell surface MHC class II molecules due to variation in invariant chain gene expression

A second and very recent set of observations relating to T-cell recognition of cell surface MHC class II molecules suggests that heterogeneity may exist in these products that cannot be accounted for simply by variation in their primary sequence. This is due to the influence of the invariant chain on the processing and transport of the class II molecule, and on the presentation of exogenous antigens.

The observation was made several years ago that MHC class II αβ dimers are associated with a third molecule, known as the invariant chain (Ii), in the cytoplasm of class II-expressing cells (Sung and Jones, 1981). This Ii polypeptide was so named because, unlike the α and β chains with which it was associated, the Ii chain did not exhibit any polymorphism. At first it was assumed that the function of the Ii chain was to assist in the assembly and transport of class II molecules to the cell surface. Consistent with this assumption was the observation that expression of the Ii gene closely parallelled expression of MHC class II genes in almost all class II-expressing cells. However, it emerged from transfection studies in which class II genes were introduced into Ii-negative cell lines, such as WEHI, that the invariant chain was not required for efficient cell surface expression of class II products. Indeed if the Ii gene was super-transfected into such a cell that was already expressing the products of transfected class II genes, no detectable benefit was observed as far as the level of MHC class II expression was concerned (Miller and Germain, 1986;

Sekaly et al., 1986). For some time this left the Ii chain as a protein without an identified function.

However, it is now apparent that the Ii chain has two roles, first of protecting class II molecules from peptide occupancy until they reach the endosomal compartment, and second of chaperoning class II molecules from the endoplasmic reticulum to the endosome. The evidence for these roles was discussed in Chapter 3. A further extrapolation of these findings is that differences have been observed between the class II molecules expressed on the surface of Ii-positive and -negative cells. These differences can be detected serologically by monoclonal antibodies (mAb), and functionally by T-cells. Using an anti-H-2A/E mAb, 40B, Peterson and Miller (1990) have noted that Ii-negative H-2A-transfected cells fail to express the 40B epitope, but H-2A transfectants which also express the Ii gene are 40B positive. An additional observation made by this group is that the H-2A-expressing, Ii-negative transfectants are unable to stimulate a strong primary alloresponse. Transfection of the Ii gene into these H-2A-positive cells renders them strongly alloimmunogenic (Miller et al., personal communication). The mechanism responsible for this Ii-mediated effect on the alloimmune response is, as yet, unexplained. It may reflect the influence of the Ii chain on the display of self peptides, or on some more general feature of MHC class II molecules. It has been noted recently that the presence of the Ii chain influences the pattern of glycosylation of cell surface class II molecules (Schaif et al., 1991). These results illustrate clearly that heterogeneity can exist in cell surface MHC class II molecules that is detectable by antibodies and by T-cells, and is determined by expression of the Ii chain. An additional possibility is that a processed form of the Ii molecule is expressed at the cell surface, and acts as an accessory molecule contributing to cell:cell avidity or to signal transduction (Jim Miller, personal communication).

These observations may have important implications for the presentation of autoantigens, and the induction of autoimmunity. As mentioned above, the expression of MHC class II and Ii genes tend to coincide in normal cells, however it may well be that the expression of these genes, which are located on different chromosomes, may not be precisely co-ordinated. Thus, during the course of a tissue-specific inflammatory response, there may be periods of time when MHC class II and Ii genes are not synchronously expressed. As outlined above, one of the roles of the Ii chain appears to be to protect the peptide-binding groove of the class II molecule from peptide occupancy until it is in the endosomal compartment of the cell. As a consequence, a relative lack of the Ii chain would be predicted to lead to the display at the cell surface of self peptides that may not have been encountered previously by T-cells, in particular during thymic ontogeny, where steady-state expression of the Ii might be expected. Under these circumstances tolerance to self antigens may be more likely to break down.

Contribution of aberrant MHC class II expression to autoimmunity

The idea was proposed several years ago that the induction of MHC class II products on the cells of inflamed tissues might be responsible for the triggering of an autoimmune response to the local tissue-specific autoantigens (Botazzo et al., 1983).

This hypothesis followed the observation that HLA-DR molecules are expressed on thyroid epithelial cells in patients with Graves' disease, and that DR-expressing epithelial cells from such a thyroid gland were able to present peptide antigen to a DR-restricted T-cell clone (Londei et al., 1984). MHC class II expression has also been detected on the β cells of pancreatic islet in a recent onset diabetic (Botazzo et al., 1985). The concept that evolved was that the T-cell repertoire may not be tolerant to some tissue-specific autoantigens which fail to reach the thymus in sufficient concentrations to cause the deletion of potentially autoreactive thymocytes. In the context of a local inflammatory response, caused by a virus with tropism for the tissue in question, MHC class II molecules may be expressed on the cells of the tissue and these cells may then present autoantigens to the trafficking T-cells that have been recruited to the site of inflammation. This model has some appeal, but some recent data about T-cell activation and tolerance pose questions about the hypothesis, and create the possibility of turning this model on its head.

T-cell antigen recognition in the absence of vital second signals leads to a state of anergy

It has emerged over the past few years that T-cell recognition does not necessarily lead to activation, but can lead to the induction of a state of profound non-responsiveness. The first observation of this kind was made with an influenza haemagglutinin (HA)-specific human T-cell clone. Overnight co-culture of this clone with the HA peptide for which it was specific, in the absence of added antigen-presenting cells, led to a state of non-responsiveness to a subsequent challenge with peptide presented by added antigen-presenting cells. The induction of tolerance was both antigen-specific, in that it required exposure to the peptide for which the clone was specific, and it was MHC class II-dependent, in that addition of anti-DR monoclonal antibody during the tolerance induction step protected the clone from being switched off (Lamb et al., 1983). Bearing in mind the fact that human T-cell clones express class II molecules, the likely interpretation of these results was that the clone was presenting peptide to itself, and that this induced non-responsiveness.

   These studies have been extended with murine T-cells, and the conditions that lead to anergy have been defined. The overall conclusions from this series of experiments are that: (1) receipt by the T-cell of signal 1 through the TcR/CD3 complex, without receipt of a second signal, leads to non-responsiveness; and (2) the genetic event underlying this state of non-responsiveness appears to be down-regulation of the interleukin-2 gene (reviewed in Jenkins et al., 1987a). This is illustrated schematically in Figure 4.3. The conditions that lead to the receipt of signal 1 without additional signalling are created if the APC are treated with the cross-linking agent 1-ethyl-3-(3-dimethylaminopropyl) carbodiimide (ECDI) (Jenkins and Schwartz, 1987), or if artificial planar membranes impregnated with class II molecules are used as surrogate antigen-presenting cells (APC) (Quill and Schwartz, 1987). The evidence for a signalling event taking place when murine T-cell clones are co-cultured with these impotent APC is that a cytoplasmic calcium flux is detectable, although protein kinase-C activation may not occur. Indeed the state of anergy can be reproduced by treating the same T-cells with a calcium ionophore which causes a calcium flux in the absence of any other signalling event (Jenkins et al., 1987b). It has become clear

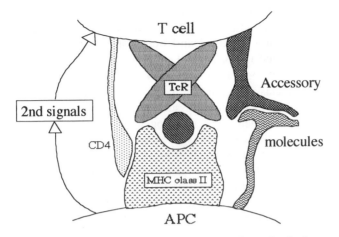

Figure 4.3 Signals required for triggering IL-2 release by T-cells. The molecular interactions involved in the activation of IL-2-secreting T-cells are shown. In addition to the specific interaction between the T-cell's receptor and its peptide/MHC ligand, and a variety of accessory molecule interactions, there is a requirement for receipt by the T-cell of 'second' or 'co-stimulatory' signals. The interaction between the T-cell surface molecule CD28 and its ligand, B7, on the APC appears to account for co-stimulation in some experimental situations.

during the past year that one of the key molecular interactions that is required for second signal generation involves B7 on the antigen-presenting cell and its two ligands on the T-cell, CD28 and CTLA-4. This is well illustrated by experiments in which tolerance induction has been prevented by the addition of antibodies specific for CD28 (Harding et al., 1992) and the capacity of an otherwise impotent cell to stimulate interleukin-2-dependent T-cell proliferation has been restored by transfection of the B7 gene (Norton et al., 1992).

The implication of these studies is that when non-professional, B7-negative, APC present antigen to T-cells, they are unable or at least inefficient at providing the crucial second signals that are required for T-cell activation. Following the observations made with murine T-cells and these artificially manipulated populations of APC the same phenomenon has been observed using normal cells, induced to express class II molecules in a variety of ways, as APC. Such cells which are constitutively negative for class II expression may be referred to as amateur APC, and have included keratinocytes and β cells of the pancreas. Co-culture of a T-cell clone that was specific for a peptide of influenza haemagglutinin in the context of DR1 and/or DR4 with HA peptide and γ-interferon (γ-IFN)-treated DR4-expressing keratinocytes (Bal et al., 1990), led to non-responsiveness of the T-cell clone. Similar findings were obtained using HLA-DR-expressing human T-cells as APC. Recognition of antigen on the surface of another T-cell, at the same concentration that led to optimal proliferation when presented by a professional APC, led to the induction of proliferative non-responsiveness by the responder T-cells (Sidhu et al., 1992). Similarly, co-culture of a pigeon cytochrome-c-specific, H-2E-restricted, mouse T-cell clone with pancreatic islet β cells expressing H-2E under the regulation of the insulin promoter led to a state of T-cell non-responsiveness (Markman et al., 1988).

The observation that specific antigen recognition on the surface of an amateur APC could lead to anergy rather than to activation of the T-cell raises a different interpretation for the consequences of class II expression on cells which do not normally have an antigen-presenting role. It could be that autoantigen recognition on amateur APC, which are unable or inefficient at providing the necessary second signals for T-cell activation, is a deliberate mechanism to protect against auto-immunity by switching potentially autoreactive T-cells off. In order to address directly the consequences of class II expression on cells which are constitutively class II negative and are located in a defined tissue, a series of MHC class II transgenic mice have been generated which express allogeneic or syngeneic class II products in the pancreas. The majority of transgene constructs have employed the rat insulin promoter (Lo et al., 1988; Starvetnick et al., 1988; Bohme et al., 1989; Miller et al., 1990) so that expression of the transgene should be targeted to the pancreas, leading to expression on the β cells of pancreatic islets. The remarkable conclusion from all of the transgenic mice of this type has been that in no case was any immune reaction observed in the class II-expressing pancreas. The first two sets of rat insulin promoter-driven class II transgenics did develop diabetes, but this turned out to be the result of a toxic effect of synthesizing high levels of MHC class II molecules, rather than from immune islet cell destruction. Using a similar approach, an MHC class I gene has been introduced under the regulation of the myelin basic protein promoter, in order to achieve stable class I expression on the surface of oligodendrocytes. This led to early death for many of the transgenic mice (Turnley et al., 1991). Once again there was no evidence for an autoimmune reaction in response to this aberrant class I expression, and the failure of myelination in these mice was thought to be the result of poisoning of oligodendrocytes due to production of high levels of MHC class I heavy chains.

The message from these transgenic experiments is clear, aberrant expression of class II molecules in the pancreas does not provoke an autoimmune, or alloimmune response. It may be argued that these experiments are not a valid test of the aberrant class II hypothesis because the transgene-encoded class II molecules are expressed from before birth, whereas the trigger to autoimmunity could be the sudden appearance of class II molecules on the cells of an inflamed tissue in adult life. Given that it is much easier to induce a state of tolerance in neonates than in adults, this could be an important difference. This argument is weakened by the lack of demonstrable tolerance to allogeneic MHC products expressed in the transgenic mice, despite their early and continuous expression. This issue may be best resolved by the introduction of class II transgenes under a tissue-specific and inducible promoter, so that class II expression can be turned on in adult life.

Although it is unclear whether the induction of MHC class II expression in tissues acts as a trigger for the onset or amplification of an autoimmune response, or has the effect of inducing a state of non-responsiveness in potentially autoreactive T-cells, there is one other source of individual variation which could be relevant to HLA-linked disease susceptibility. It is possible that polymorphism exists in the regulatory regions of MHC class II genes, leading to variation in the inducibility of these genes. Whether class II induction contributes to, or protects from autoimmunity, individual variation in the regulation of class II gene expression by cytokines could lead to quantitative or even qualitative differences in immune reactivity. This possibility is currently being investigated.

References

Bakke, O. and Dobberstein, B. (1990). MHC class II-associated invariant chain contains a sorting signal for endosomal compartments. *Cell* **63**: 707–716.

Bal, V., McIndoe, A., Denton, G. et al. (1990). Antigen presentation by keratinocytes induces tolerance in human T cells. *Euro. J. Immunol.* **20**: 1893–1897.

Beck, B.N., Frelinger, J.G., Shigeta, M. et al. (1982). T cell clones specific for hybrid I-A molecules. Discrimination with monoclonal anti-I-Ak antibodies. *J. Exp. Med.* **156**: 1186–1193.

Bohme, J., Haskins, K., Stecha, P. et al. (1989). Transgenic mice with I-A on islet cells are normoglycemic but immunologically intolerant. *Science* **244**: 1179–1183.

Bottazzo, G.F., Pujol-Borrell, R. and Hanafusa, T. (1983). Role of aberrant HLA-DR expression and antigen presentation in induction of enodcrine autoimmunity. *Lancet* **2**: 1115–1119.

Bottazzo, G.F., Dean, B.M., McNally, J.M. et al. (1985). In situ characterization of autoimmune phenomena and expression of HLA molecules in the pancreas in diabetes mellitus. *N. Engl. J. Med.* **313**: 353–360.

Braunstein, N.S. and Germain, R.N. (1987). Allele-specific control of Ia molecule surface expression and conformation: implications for a model Ia structure–function relationship. *Proc. Natl Acad. Sci. USA* **84**: 2921–2924.

Harding, F., McArthur, J., Gross, J. et al. (1992). CD28-mediated signalling co-stimulates murine T cells and prevents induction of anergy in T-cell clones. *Nature* **356**: 607–609.

Jenkins, M.K. and Schwartz, R.H. (1987). Antigen presentation by chemically modified splenocytes induces antigen-specific T cell unresponsiveness in vitro and in vivo. *J. Exp. Med.* **165**: 3704–3713.

Jenkins, M.K., Pardoll, M.D., Mizuguchi, J. et al. (1987a). T-cell unresponsiveness in vivo and in vitro; fine specificity of induction and molecular characterization of the unresponsive state. *Immunol. Rev.* **95**: 113–135.

Jenkins, M.K., Pardoll, D.M., Mizuguchi, J. et al. (1987b). Molecular events in the induction of a nonresponsive state in interleukin 2-producing helper T-lymphocyte clones. *Proc. Natl Acad. Sci. USA* **84**: 1–6.

Kwok, W.W., Schwarz, D., Nepom, B.S. et al. (1988). HLA-DQ molecules form $\alpha\beta$ heterodimers of mixed allotype. *J. Immunol.* **141**: 3123–3127.

Lamb, J.R., Skidmore, B.J. and Green, N. (1983). Induction of tolerance in influenza virus-immune T lymphocyte clones with synthetic peptides of influenza haemagglutinin. *J. Exp. Med.* **157**: 1434.

Lechler, R.I. (1988). MHC class II molecular structure – permitted pairs? *Immunol. Today* **9**: 76–78.

Lo, D., Burkly, L.C., Widera, G. et al. (1988). Diabetes and tolerance in transgenic mice expressing class II molecules in pancreatic beta cells. *Cell* **53**: 159–168.

Londei, M., Lamb, J.R., Bottazzo, G.F. et al. (1984). Epithelial cells expressing aberrant MHC class II determinants can present antigen to cloned human T cells. *Nature* **312**: 639–610.

Lotteau, V., Teyton, L., Burroughs, D. et al. (1987). A novel HLA class II molecule (DRαDQβ) created by mismatched isotype pairing. *Nature* **329**: 339–341.

Lotteau, V., Sands, J., Teyton, L. et al. (1989). Modulation of HLA class II antigen expression of sense and antisense DRa cDNA. *J. Exp. Med.* **169**: 351–356.

Markman, J., Lo, D., Naji, A. et al. (1988). Antigen-presenting function of class II MHC-expressing pancreatic beta cells. *Nature* **336**: 476–479.

Miller, J., Daitch, L., Rath, S. et al. (1990). Tissue-specific expression of allogeneic class II MHC molecules induces neither tissue rejection nor clonal inactivation of alloreactive T cells. *J. Immunol.* **144**: 334–341.

Norton, S., Zuckerman, L., Urdahl, R. et al. (1992). The CD28 ligand, B7, enhances IL-2 production by providing a costimulatory signal to T cells. *J. Immunol.* **149**: 1556–1562.

Peterson, M. and Miller, J. (1990). Invariant chain influences the immunological recognition of MHC class II molecules. *Nature* **345**: 172–174.

Quill, H. and Schwartz, R.H. (1987). Stimulation of normal inducer T cell clones with antigen presented by purified Ia molecules in planar lipid membranes: specific induction of a long-lived state of proliferative non-responsiveness. *J. Immunol.* **138**: 3704–3712.

Ruberti, G., Sellins, K.S., Hill, C.M. et al. (1991). Presentation of antigen by mixed isotype class II molecules in normal H-2d mice. *J. Exp. Med.* **175**: 157–162.

Sant, A.J. and Germain, R.N. (1989). Intracellular competition for component chains determines class II MHC cell surface phenotype. *Cell* **57**: 797–805.

Schaiff, W.T., Hruska, K.A. and Bono, C. (1991). Invariant chain influences post-translational processing of HLA-DR molecules. *J. Immunol.* **147**: 603–608.

Sekaly, R.P., Tonnelle, C., Strubin, M. et al. (1986). Cell surface expression of class II histocompatibility antigens occurs in the absence of the invariant chain. *J. Exp. Med.* **164**: 1490–1504.

Starvetnick, N., Liggitt, D. and Pitts, S.L. (1988). Insulin-dependent diabetes mellitus induced in transgenic mice by ectopic expression of class II MHC and interferon-gamma. *Cell* **52**: 773–781.

Sung, E. and Jones, P.P. (1981). The invariant chain of murine Ia antigens: its glycosylation, abundance, and subcellular localization. *Mol. Immunol.* **18**: 899–913.

Turnley, A.M., Morahan, G., Okano, H. et al. (1991). Dysmyelination in transgenic mice resulting from expression of class I histocompatibility molecules in oligodendrocytes. *Nature* **353**: 566–569.

CHAPTER 5
Mechanisms of HLA and disease associations

Robert Lechler
Department of Immunology
Royal Postgraduate Medical School
London, UK

In the first part of this book, the basic principles underlying MHC-restricted recognition of antigens by T-cells were outlined. These included extensive reference to the phenomenon of MHC-determined variation in immune responsiveness. Armed with these concepts, this chapter undertakes a discussion of the mechanisms underlying the association between the inheritance of particular MHC alleles and disease susceptibility, making references to some of the well-studied animal models of autoimmune disease.

One important distinction to make before considering the mechanisms responsible for an individual disease association is between autoimmune, immune complex-mediated and non-immune diseases. For these purposes autoimmune diseases are defined as those diseases whose pathogenesis results from the direct effects of a specific immune response (either an autoantibody, or an autoreactive T-cell response) against host tissues. A classical example of an autoimmune disease that fits this definition is anti-glomerular basement membrane (anti-GBM) disease, otherwise known as Goodpasture's syndrome. Tissue damage in this condition does appear to be caused by the circulating anti-GBM antibody, which can be detected with a characteristic pattern of linear deposition on the renal glomerular, and the pulmonary alveolar basement membranes. This contrasts with an immune complex disease such as systemic lupus erythematosus (SLE). Autoantibodies, in this case against double-stranded DNA, are also a feature of SLE, however, the pathogenicity of the anti-DNA antibodies in this disease is a point of continuing debate. SLE is an archetypal immune complex-mediated disease, and the systemic vasculitis that can affect multiple sites in this condition appears to be the result of the deposition, or the in situ formation, of insoluble immune complexes. Some of these may be DNA:anti-DNA complexes. The third category of HLA-associated diseases do not have any known immune component in their pathogenesis. Narcolepsy is a classical example of this

HLA and Disease
ISBN 0–12–440320–4

Table 5.1   Some examples of HLA-associated diseases, divided according to their pathogenetic mechanism

Group	Disease	HLA marker
No autoimmune aetiology	21-Hydroxylase deficiency	Deletion of the 21-OH B gene (Bw47)[a]
	Idiopathic haemochromatosis	A3
Autoimmune aetiology	Ankylosing spondylitis	B27
	Rheumatoid arthritis	DR4Dw4/14, DR1
	Coeliac disease	B8 DR3 DQw2
	Insulin-dependent diabetes mellitus	DR3,4 DQw7/8
	Multiple sclerosis (in Caucasians)	DRw15 DQw6
	Goodpasture's syndrome	DRw15 DQw6
Unknown aetiology	Narcolepsy	DRw15

[a] The 21-OH B deletion is in linkage disequilibrium with Bw47

kind of disease, in that a strong association has been documented with HLA-DRw15 (Juji et al., 1983), but there is little to suggest an autoimmune or immune complex-mediated pathogenesis in this condition. These are clearly important distinctions to make because they will help in the interpretation of HLA associations. Some of the well-characterized HLA-associated diseases, divided according to the mechanisms that are thought to underlie their pathogenesis, are presented in Table 5.1.

Ir gene effects and disease susceptibility

As described in detail in Chapter 3, many experimental examples have been documented of genetically determined variation in immune responsiveness to individual antigenic determinants that map to the MHC. The three major mechanisms underlying this MHC-linked variation were also reviewed in Chapter 3, and were: (1) determinant selection; (2) holes in the T-cell repertoire; and (3) T-cell-mediated suppression. Experimental evidence implicating these mechanisms in two animal models of autoimmune disease will be discussed below.

Experimental allergic encephalomyelitis

This is a demyelinating disease which can be induced in several animal strains, and causes varying degrees of paralysis or even death. It is characterized by infiltration of the white matter of the central nervous system (CNS) by mononuclear cells, and is clearly immunologically mediated. This disease is induced by the injection of the CNS autoantigen myelin basic protein (MBP). The route of immunization in most of these experimental models is intradermal and the induction of immunity requires the use of a potent adjuvant such as complete Freund's adjuvant. Models of the disease have been described in rabbits (Stuart and Krikorian, 1928), mice (Olitsky and Yager, 1949), rats and guinea-pigs (Paterson, 1976). The reason that so much research effort has been channelled into the study of experimental allergic encephalomyelitis (EAE) is because it is one of the most well-characterized experimental models of the human demyelinating disease multiple sclerosis (MS).

In the mouse model of EAE it is clear that genetic factors control susceptibility to developing an autoimmune response. The best defined of these genetic factors is the possession of certain MHC class II H-2A alleles. Two of these, namely H-2A^s and H-2A^u, have been studied in detail, and the precise specificity of autoimmune T-cells have been determined (Zamvil et al., 1988). As befits this MHC class II association, CD4$^+$ T-cells are the major disease-inducing population in EAE. Thus, anti-CD4 antibodies were able to prevent disease in mice and rats (Brostoff and Mason, 1984; Waldor et al., 1985). Furthermore, CD4$^+$, MBP-specific T-cell clones were able to induce EAE following transfer to naive recipient mice (Zamvil et al., 1985). In addition, the injection of anti-MHC class II antibodies was able to confer protection from EAE (Steinman et al., 1983).

There are three sets of observations regarding EAE that relate to the issue of MHC and disease associations. The first is that for both of the H-2A types which cause disease susceptibility, a distinct peptide specificity has been defined in the disease-mediating MBP-specific T-cells. For the H-2A^s-bearing mice, the T-cell response appears to be almost entirely directed against an MBP sequence comprising amino-acid residues 89–101 (Sakai et al., 1988). In contrast, the specificity of T-cells from H-2A^u-expressing mice is for the N-terminal region of MBP between residues 1 and 11 (Zamvil et al., 1988). This provides a clear example of the influence of MHC polymorphism on T-cell specificity. These findings have been further explored by examining the efficiency of binding of these peptides of MBP to the H-2A^s and H-2A^u molecules. As might be expected, the 1–11 peptide bound efficiently to H-2A^u, and this binding could not be significantly inhibited by addition of a large molar excess of the H-2A^s-restricted 89–101 peptide (Wraith et al., 1989). Although these results illustrate the influence of H-2A polymorphism on the specificity of an autoimmune response, it remains unclear whether the fact that other H-2A types are not associated with susceptibility to EAE is because they do not bind and present available peptides of MBP efficiently. This would be the case if determinant selection was the sole explanation for the MHC association. Alternatively H-2A^s- and H-2A^u-associated disease susceptibility may reflect the influence of these MHC products on the selection of the T-cell repertoire, or on the induction of suppressor T-cells.

A second series of important observations relating to the pathogenesis of EAE have focused attention on T-cell receptor usage in MBP-specific T-cells in autoimmune animals. The remarkable finding was that the large majority of MBP-reactive T-cell clones isolated from autoimmune mice and rats used the same Vβ gene segment, and one of two Vα segments (Bβ8.2 and Vα2 or 4) (Zamvil et al., 1988; Acha-Orbea et al., 1989). Given the proportion of mouse peripheral T-cells which express these V gene segments, the frequency of T-cells expressing these particular combinations of Vβ8.2 and Vα2 or 4 should be in the region of 1 in 1000, assuming a random αβ chain association. It is particularly surprising that the same receptor should appear in MBP-immune T-cells from the rat as well as the mouse (Heber-Katz and Acha-Orbea, 1989). The MBP peptide specificity of the T-cells from the two species is quite different, and the degree of sequence homology between the rat and mouse MHC class II restriction elements is only of the order of 80%. Although these observations are difficult to explain, they do suggest that T-cell repertoire selection is influential in the aetiology of this disease. It is interesting to note that preferential usage of the Vα11 gene segment has been recently reported in T-cells isolated from the cerebrospinal fluid of MS patients (Oksenberg et al., 1990).

The third set of data relating to the autoimmune response mediating EAE suggests that suppressor T-cells can play an important role in regulating anti-MBP immunity. It was noted several years ago that if guinea-pigs were injected *intravenously* with MBP prior to intradermal immunization with Freund's adjuvant, the animals were protected from the development of disease. Furthermore, T-cells from these pre-treated animals conferred protection from EAE when transferred to naive syngeneic recipients (Arnon, 1981). This illustrates that autoimmunity of this kind is susceptible to T-cell regulation. As yet there is no evidence that regulation of this sort plays a role in the protection of non-susceptible animals from developing EAE.

The conclusion that can be drawn about the MHC association with EAE from these studies is that all three of the mechanisms proposed in Chapter 3, and outlined at the start of this chapter, could contribute to MHC-linked susceptibility to anti-MBP autoimmunity. Further elucidation of the underlying mechanisms may be furnished by carefully designed transgenic mouse experiments.

The non-obese diabetic mouse

In the same way that EAE serves as a model for the human disease MS, the non-obese diabetic (NOD) mouse serves as an experimental model of human insulin-dependent diabetes. Diabetes in these mice is characterized by autoimmune insulitis and destruction of pancreatic β cells. Unlike EAE, diabetes in this mouse strain occurs spontaneously; in common with EAE it is clear that more than one genetic locus is responsible for disease susceptibility. One of the key susceptibility genes for the development of disease in NOD mice is a unique allele of the Ab gene, known as Ab[NOD] (Acha-Orbea and McDevitt, 1987). This Ab allele is accompanied by an entirely normal Aa[d] gene. It is of particular interest that the polypeptide encoded by the Ab[NOD] gene lacks the negatively charged aspartic acid at position 57. Lack of aspartic acid at this position in the human homologue of Aβ, DQβ, appears to be associated with susceptibility to insulin-dependent diabetes in man (Todd et al., 1987). The other feature of the class II region of NOD mice is a defect in the H-2E genes that encode the second mouse class II product, so that no H-2E molecule is expressed.

Investigation of the mechanisms responsible for the MHC and disease association in this model is hampered by the fact that the pancreatic autoantigen(s) has not been defined. It is not possible therefore to grow disease-mediating T-cells, and explore their specificity or T-cell receptor gene usage. None the less a series of genetic and immunological interventions have led to protection from the onset of disease and these results provide clues about the contribution of the MHC haplotype to this autoimmune reaction. There is evidence to suggest that both the possession of the Ab[NOD] gene and the lack of H-2E expression may contribute to the development of diabetes in these mice. The most informative experiments in this area have involved the production of transgenic mice into which have been transferred genes encoding normal or mutated H-2A and wild-type H-2E molecules. Nishimoto and colleagues (1987) observed that the introduction of an H-2E transgene into NOD mice prevented the development of insulitis. This result argues strongly that the lack of H-2E expression is an important factor in the tendency of these mice to autoimmune insulitis. The recent results of Slattery et al. (1990), Nishimoto et al. (1987) and Lund et al. (1990) provide evidence that disease susceptibility in NOD mice can be attenuated or abolished by introduction of H-2A transgenes. Protection was achieved by expression of wild-type H-2A^k (Slattery), H-2A^k with serine rather than the charged aspartic acid at position 57 of the H-2Aβ chain (Nishimoto) (as discussed above, it has been suggested that a charged residue in DQ and H-2A β chains at this position confers protection from disease), and by expression of H-2A with proline rather than histidine at position 56 in the β chain (Lund). In addition to having an uncharged residue at position 57, the Aβ^{NOD} chain is unique in having histidine at position 56. Despite the fact that the A$\beta^{NOD-56\ pro}$ chain retained the uncharged serine at position 57 this modified Aβ chain still conferred protection, further emphasizing that the contribution of MHC class II genes to susceptibility to diabetes cannot be entirely accounted for by polymorphism at position 57 in DQ and H-2A β chains.

The protective effects of introducing a wild-type H-2E gene, or mutated H-2Ab genes into NOD mice shed some light on the probable mechanisms of susceptibility to autoimmune destruction of pancreatic β cells. The most likely explanation for these effects is that the introduction of additional class II genes alters the expressed T-cell repertoire in the transgenic mice. This could be the result of intrathymic deletion of potentially autoreactive T-cells due to reactivity of such cells with the additional expressed class II products, or could be the result of selection of regulatory suppressor T-cells that prevent the development of disease in the transgenic animals. Thus, it is possible that all three of the major mechanisms of Ir gene effects contribute to susceptibility to diabetes in NOD mice, and susceptibility to demyelination in mice that develop EAE.

Molecular mimicry

It has long been known that cross-reactions between microbial antigens and auto-antigens can arise, and can lead to an autoimmune response. Two of the earliest examples of this kind of molecular mimicry to be defined were between *Trypanosoma cruzi* and Streptococcal antigens and the myocardium, giving rise to the manifestations of Chagas' disease and rheumatic fever (Williams, 1983).

A more contentious hypothesis was put forward several years ago to account for the pathogenesis of the rheumatological disease, ankylosing spondylitis. Two groups reported that antibodies raised against the gut pathogen *Klebsiella* reacted with lymphocytes from HLA-B27-positive patients with ankylosing spondylitis (Ebringer, 1979; Seager et al., 1979). They also observed that anti-B27 antibodies cross-reacted with various enterobacteria, including *Klebsiella*. This was followed up by the finding that monoclonal antibodies raised against B27 also recognized antigens expressed by *Klebsiella*, *Salmonella*, *Shigella*, and *Yersinia* organisms. The significance of these cross-reactions is that these organisms are the very ones that can provoke reactive arthritis in B27-positive individuals.

There are, however, a number of problems with this hypothesis that are responsible for its failure to achieve general acceptance. At a conceptual level it is unclear why this kind of cross-reaction should give rise to a disease that is confined, in most cases to the joints. Furthermore, other groups have failed to reproduce these original observations in other groups of patients (Archer, 1981). Indeed in one recent study, antibodies specific for a shared determinant carried by HLA-B27 and by a strain of

Klebsiella were found with equal frequency in patients and controls (Tsuchiya et al., 1989). This is discussed in more detail in Chapter 7.

Another set of molecules that have received considerable attention in recent years, because of the possibility of cross-reactivity between pathogen and host homologues, are the heat shock proteins. These molecules are highly conserved across a remarkably wide range of organisms, from bacteria to man. It has been postulated that the induction of T-cell immunity against a bacterial or a mycobacterial heat shock protein could lead to cross-reactive recognition of autologous heat shock proteins (Kaufman et al., 1991). There is every reason to think that either the initial response to the foreign antigen, or the cross-reaction on the autoantigen, will be under HLA-linked immune response gene control.

MHC class I and II molecules as receptors for viruses and drugs

The mechanism by which many viruses enter cells involves attachment to cell surface glycoproteins, followed by fusion of their membranes with the cell's plasma membrane either at the cell surface or after endocytosis. Such cellular receptor proteins have to be glycoproteins that recycle or which undergo endocytosis after virus-induced cross-linking. HLA antigens fit these criteria. Some of the documented molecules that are known to be involved in viral entry into cells are the C3d receptor for the Epstein–Barr virus (Jonsson et al., 1982), and the CD4 molecule for the HIV-1 virus (Dalgleish et al., 1984). Three viruses have been shown to adhere specifically to mouse or human MHC molecules. The Semliki forest virus and adenovirus type 2 bind to MHC class I (Helenius et al., 1982; Signas et al., 1982) and the lactate dehydrogenase virus to class II molecules (Inada and Mims, 1984). It is possible that some viruses actually enter cells by forming specific attachments to HLA antigens. This would create the possibility of some HLA types conferring resistance to particular viruses. However, this would lead to a strong selective advantage for mutant viruses that escaped from this allelic restriction. Given that there is an enormous difference in the generation times of viruses and humans it is difficult to see how viral glycoproteins and HLA molecules could exist in a stable state of balanced polymorphism.

Roles of non-HLA genes within the human MHC

One of the important implications of the strong linkage disequilibrium that characterizes the MHC region is that caution must always be exercised when interpreting a correlation between a raised frequency of an HLA allelic marker and a human disease. As discussed in detail (and referenced) in Chapters 1, 2, and 9 of this book, many genes are present within the MHC in addition to those that encode the HLA antigens. Some of these have already been characterized, and include genes that encode proteins with obvious relevance to the immune system. These include genes in the class III region that encode the complement components C2, C4, and factor B, the tumour necrosis factor (TNF)-A and -B genes and the genes for the heat shock protein, Hsp-70. More recently genes encoding peptide transporters and proteasome units have been identified within the class II region. However, this may be regarded as only the tip of the iceberg, and there are a large number of other genes within the MHC which will be characterized during the next few years. It remains to be seen whether these additional genes encode products which influence, or are directly involved in the immune system, and whether they exhibit significant polymorphism. None the less, the possibility exists that the true susceptibility gene underlying some HLA-associated diseases may be one of these non-HLA genes. The apparent HLA association may reflect the fact that tight linkage disequilibrium exists between allelic variants of the non-HLA and the HLA genes.

Returning to two of the recently defined non-HLA genes in the MHC region, namely the genes encoding TNFα and β, and the Hsp-70 genes, both of these have tantalizing possible links with the immune response. TNFβ is one of the soluble factors which can induce and/or enhance the expression of MHC class II genes in some cell types (Arenzana-Scisdedos et al., 1988). It has already been established that there is restriction fragment length polymorphism at this locus (Partanen and Koskimies, 1988; Jacob et al., 1990); it is not yet known whether this reflects coding region or regulatory sequence variation which could, in turn, lead to functional differences in the induction of the TNF-B gene or in its efficiency in inducing class II expression. Given the key role that class II molecules play in T-cell immune responses, variation in the effects of TNF could exert a strong influence on autoimmunity. Of particular relevance to this suggestion is the observation that quantitative variation in the expression of MHC class II molecules can have profound effects on T-cell responses. This has been demonstrated using class II-expressing transfectants (Lechler et al., 1985), and is reviewed by Janeway (1985). As discussed in Chapter 4, the induction of class II molecules on non-bone marrow-derived cells in solid organs, is predicted to influence the course of an autoimmune response. Whether this class II induction has an amplifying or a dampening effect on a local autoimmune reaction remains a point of debate. None the less individual variation in the inducibility of class II molecules in tissues, related to allelic variation in TNF genes, could very well act as an important contributor to disease susceptibility.

In a similar manner, allelic variation in the Hsp-70 gene could affect T-cell immunity. Preliminary evidence exists to suggest that this stress protein plays a role in the intra-cellular handling of internalized antigens (Parham, 1990), and poly-morphisms have been defined (Milner and Campbell, 1990). The relevance of these genes, and the many others that are currently being characterized within the HLA region, to HLA and disease associations will be discussed in more detail in Chapter 9.

References

Acha-Orbea, H., Steinman, L. and McDevitt, H. (1989). T cell receptors in murine autoimmune diseases. *Ann. Rev. Immunol.* **7**: 371–405.

Bottazzo, G., Pujol-Borrell, R. and Hanafusa, T. (1983). Role of aberrant HLA-DR expression and antigen presentation in induction of endocrine autoimmunity. *Lancet* **2**: 1115–1119.

Bottazzo, G., Dean, B., McNally, J. et al. (1985). In situ characterization of autoimmune phenomena and expression of HLA molecules in the pancreas in diabetes mellitus. *N. Engl. J. Med.* **313**: 353–360.

Brostoff, S. and Mason, D. (1984). Experimental allergic encephalomyeitis: successful treatment in vivo with a monoclonal antibody that recognizes T helper cells. *J. Immunol.* **133**: 1938–1942.

Acha-Orbea, H. and McDevitt, H.O. (1987). The first external domain of the nonobese diabetic mouse class II I-A beta chain is unique. *Proc. Natl. Acad. Sci. USA* **84**: 2435–2439.

Archer, J.R. (1981). Search for cross-reactivity between HLA B27 associated and Klebsiellapneumoniac. *Ann Rheum. Dis.* **40**: 400–403.

Arenzana-Scisdedos, F., Mogensen, S.C., Vuillier, F. et al. (1988). Autocrine secretion of tumor necrosis factor under the influence of interferon-gamma amplifies HLA-DR gene induction in human monocytes. *Proc. Natl. Acad. Sci. USA* **85**: 6087–6091.

Arnon, R. (1981). Experimental allergic encephalomyelitis-susceptibility and suppression. *Immunol. Rev.* **55**: 5–30.

Castano, L. and Eisenbarth, G. (1990). Type-1 diabetes: a chronic autoimmune disease of human, mouse, and rat. *Ann. Rev. Immunol.* **8**: 647–679.

Dalgleish, A., Beverley, P., Clapham, P. et al. (1984). The CD4(T4) antigen is an essential component of the receptor for AIDS retrovirus. *Nature* **312**: 763–767.

Dyson, P., Knight, A., Fairchild, S. et al. (1991). Genes encoding ligands for deletion of Vβ11 T cells cosegregate with mammary tumour virus genomes. *Nature* **349**: 530–531.

Ebringer, A. (1979). Ankylosing spondylitis, immune-response-genes and molecular mimicry. *Lancet* **1**: 1186 (letter).

Frankel, W., Rudy, C., Coffin, J. et al. (1991). Linkage of MIs genes to endogenous mammary tumour viruses of inbred mice. *Nature* **349**: 526–527.

Heber-Katz, E. and Acha-Orbea, H. (1989). The V-region disease hypothesis: evidence from autoimmune encephalomyelitis. *Immunol. Today* **10**: 164–169.

Helenius, A., Morein, B., Fries, E. et al. (1982). Human (HLA-A and HLA-B) and murine (H-2K and H-2C) histocompatibility antigens are cell surface receptors for Semliki Forest virus. *Proc. Natl. Acad. Sci. USA* **75**: 3846–3850.

Jacob, C., Fronek, Z., Lewis, G. et al. (1990). Heritable major histocompatibility complex class II-associated differences in production of tumour necrosis factor α: relevance to systemic lupus erythematosus. *Proc. Natl Acad. Sci. USA* **87**: 1233–1237.

Jonsson, V., Wells, A. and Klein, G. (1982). Receptors for the complement C3d component and the Epstein–Barr virus are quantitatively co-expressed on a series of B cell lines and their derived somatic cell hybrids. *Cell Immunol.* **72**: 263–276.

Juji, T., Satake, M., Honda, Y. et al (1983). HLA antigens in Japanese patients with narcolepsy: all patients were DR2 positive. *Tissue Antigens* **24**: 316–319.

Kaufmann, S.H., Schoel, B., van Embden, D. et al. (1991). Heat-shock protein 60: implications for pathogenesis of and protection against bacterial infections. *Immunol. Rev.* **121**: 67–90.

Lechler, R.I. (1985) Qualitative and quantitative studies of antigen-presenting cell function by using I-A-expressing L cells. *J. Immunol.* **135**: 2914–2922.

Lund, T., O'Reilly, L., Hutchings, P. et al. (1990). Prevention of insulin-dependent diabetes mellitus in non-obese diabetic mice by transgenes encoding modified I-A β-chain or normal I-E α-chain. *Nature* **345**: 727–729.

Marrack, P., Kushnir, E. and Kappler, J. (1991). A maternally inherited superantigen encoded by a mammary tumour virus. *Nature* **349**: 524–525.

Milner, C.M. and Campbell, R.D. (1990). Structure and expression of the three MHC-linked HSP70 genes. *Immunogenetics* **32**: 242–251.

Miyazaki, T., Uno, M., Kikutani, H. et al. (1990). Direct evidence for the contribution of the unique I-A^NOD to the development of insulinitis in non-obese diabetic mice. *Nature* **345**: 722–724.

Nishimoto, H., Kikurani, H., Yamamura, K. et al. (1987). Prevention of autoimmune insulitis by expression of I-E molecules in NOD mice. *Nature* **328**: 432–434.

Okensenberg, J.R., Stuart, S. Begovich, A.B., et al. (1990) Limited heterogeneity of rearranged T-cell receptor V alpha transcripts in brains of multiple sclerosis patients. *Nature* **353**: 94.

Olitsky, P. and Yager, R. (1949). Experimental disseminated encephalomyelitis in white mice. *J. Exp. Med.* **90**: 213–113.

Patarnen, J. and Koskimies, S. (1988). Low degree of DNA polymorphism in the HLA-linked lymphotoxin (Tumour Necrosis Factor β) gene. *Scand. J. Immunol.* **28**: 313–316.

Paterson, P. (1976). Experimental allergic encephalomyelitis and autoimmune disease. *Adv. Immunol.* **5**: 131–153.

Rivers, T. and Schwentker, F. (1935). Encephalomyelitis accompanied by myelin destruction experimentally produced in monkeys. *J. Exp. Med.* **61**: 689–702.

Sakai, K., Sinha, A., Mitchell, D. et al. (1988). Involvement of distinct T cell receptors in the autoimmune encephalitogenic response to nested epitopes of myelin basic protein. *Proc. Natl Acad. Sci. USA* **85**: 8608–8612.

Scott, C. and Steinman, L. (1990). The T lymphocyte in experimental allergic encephalomyelitis. *Ann. Rev. Immunol.* **8**: 579–621.

Seager, K., Bashir, H.V., Geczy, A.F. et al. (1979). Evidence for a specific B27-associated cell surface marker on lymphocytes of patients with ankylosing spondylitis. *Nature* **277**: 68–70.

Signas, C., Katze, M., Persson, H. et al. (1982). An adenovirus glycoprotein binds heavy chains of class I transplantation antigens from man and mouse. *Nature* **299**: 175–178.

Slattery, R., Kjer-Nielsen, L., Allison, J. et al. (1990). Prevention of diabetes in non-obese diabetic I-A^k transgenic mice. *Nature* **345**: 724–727.

Steinman, L., Solomon, D., Zamvil, S. et al. (1983). Prevention of EAE with anti I-A antibody: decreased accumulation of radiolabelled lymphocytes in the central nervous system. *J. Neuroimmunol.* **5**: 91–97.

Stuart, G. and Krikorian, K. (1928). The neuroparalytic accidents of anti-rabies treatment. *Ann. Trop. Med. Parasitol.* **22**: 327–377.

Todd, J.A., Bell, J.I. and McDevitt, H.O. (1987). HLA-DQ beta gene contributes to susceptibility and resistance to insulin-dependent diabetes mellitus. *Nature* **329**: 599–604.

Todd, J., Fukui, Y. and Kitagawa, T. (1990). The A3 allele of the HLA-DQA1 locus is associated with susceptibility to type I diabetes in Japanese. *Proc. Natl Acad. Sci. USA* **87**: 1094–1098.

Tsuchiya, N., Husby, G., and Williams, R.C. (1989). Studies of humoral and cell-mediated immunity to peptides shared by HLA-B27.1 and *Klebsiella pneumoniae* nitorgenase in ankylosing spondylitis. *Clin. Exp. Immunol.* **76**: 354–360.

Turnley, A., Morahan, G., Okano, H. et al. (1991). Dysmyelination in transgenic mice resulting from expression of class I histocompatibility molecules in oligodendrocytes. *Nature* **353**: 566–567.

Waldor, M., Sriram, S., Hardy, R. et al. (1985). Reversal of experimental allergic encephalomyelitis with a monoclonal antibody to a T cell subset marker (L3T4). *Science* **227**: 415–417.

Williams, R. (1983). Rheumatic fever and the streptococcus. *Am. J. Med.* **75**: 727–730.

Woodlan, D., Happ, M., Gollob, K. et al. (1991). An endogenous retrovirus mediating deletion of αβ T cells? *Nature* **349**: 528–529.

Wraith, D., McDevitt, H., Steinman, L. and Acha-Orbea, H. (1989). T-cell recognition as the target for immune intervention in autoimmune disease. *Cell* **57**: 709–715.

Zamvil, S.S., Mitchell, D.J., Powell, M.B. et al. (1988). Multiple discrete encephalitogenic epitopes of the autoantigen myelin basic protein include a determinant for I-E class II-restricted T cells. *J. Exp. Med.* **168**: 1181–1186.

Zamvil, S., Nelson, P., Trotter, J. et al. (1985). T cell clones specific for myelin basic protein induce chronic relapsing EAE and demyelination. *Nature* **317**: 355–358.

Zamvil, S., Nelson, P., Mitchell, D. et al. (1985). Encephalitogenic T cell clones specific for myelin basic protein: an unusual bias in antigen presentation. *J. Exp. Med.* **162**: 2107–2124.

CHAPTER 6

Design and interpretation of studies of the major histocompatibility complex in disease

Philip Dyer and Anthony Warrens

*Department of Medical Genetics, University of Manchester, Manchester, UK;
Department of Immunology, Royal Postgraduate Medical School,
London, UK*

Introduction

Using serological methods, the first demonstration of an association between an HLA antigen and a well-defined human disease came in 1973 when it was shown that about 95% of patients with ankylosing spondylitis typed for HL-Aw27 (now HLA-B27) contrasting with a frequency of about 5% in normal persons (Brewerton et al., 1973; Schlosstein et al., 1973). This pioneering work led to a rapid expansion in the number of studies seeking to establish associations between HLA antigens and diseases. However, these early studies suffered from poorly defined patient populations, the ability to type for only a few of the currently known HLA antigens, small numbers of patients and inadequate controls. None the less, some remarkable associations were detected, and more recent studies have confirmed and extended much of the early data on HLA and disease associations.

Despite the enormous literature that has already accumulated in the field of HLA and disease associations, we are now in what promises to be a particularly productive period for studying the associations between HLA antigens and disease for three reasons. First, the advances in technology, particularly in recombinant DNA techniques, have made the definition of HLA alleles considerably more precise, rapid and efficient. Second, understanding of how the structures of MHC molecules subserve their functions has progressed rapidly since the three-dimensional structure of HLA-A2 was solved in 1987 (Bjorkman et al., 1987). This enables observations of associations to be interpreted mechanistically. Third, the discovery of multiple genes

HLA and Disease
ISBN 0–12–440320–4

within the HLA region that encode proteins other that HLA antigens opens up the possibility that non-HLA genes, in linkage with HLA loci, may be the true susceptibility genes for some diseases. There is still much to be discovered in this area and there is considerable scope for intelligently designed studies. The aim of this chapter is to facilitate such work. It hardly needs to be stated that studies in this field require careful planning in order to maximize the likelihood of acquiring statistically significant results. Not only are poorly defined studies wasteful of time, but the techniques used to define HLA types and HLA gene polymorphisms are costly and use reagents that are in limited supply. The most productive studies result from open and full collaboration between scientists and clinicians, and between centres with shared interests.

Study design and execution

Need for a study

The impetus for an HLA and disease study usually comes from a clinician with access to a patient group. In the first instance, reference texts should be consulted to ascertain whether previous studies in a similar patient group have been documented; currently the text by Tiwari and Terasaki contains the most comprehensive list even though it was published in 1985. A literature search using one of the established computerized databases of published work can also be performed quite quickly.

The criteria for proceeding will be met if no previous such study is published, if the proposed study will use more refined techniques for defining HLA alleles or will detect polymorphisms of non-HLA genes within the HLA region, if previous studies were only of small groups of patients, if previous studies were on poorly characterized patients, or if new clinical data relating to disease diagnosis has recently become available. This last point is illustrated when a single disease can be divided into two or more subgroups due to advances in clinical diagnostic criteria. This has occurred in the systemic vasculitides, for example, following the development of new autoantibody tests.

Definition of patient groups

It is essential to set out clearly agreed criteria for inclusion of patients in any study. This will avoid unnecessary testing of patients' blood samples and collation of irrelevant data. It is often the case that reviewing patients during a study leads to alteration of diagnoses.

The prevalence of the disease under consideration usually determines the number of patients to be included in the study. For the more common diseases, patient samples can be obtained quickly; for the rarer diseases, sampling over a wide geographical area may be necessary. A further consideration is the need to include sufficient study participants to satisfy the needs of the statistical tests which are essential if conclusive results are to be obtained. As a general rule, at least 50 patients must be included in a study. However, when studying a rare disease, smaller patient numbers may be sufficient, particularly if a strong association with an HLA antigen is found. Admittance of patients to a study should be the responsibility of the participating clinician.

It is usual to set study commencement and end times; this helps laboratory staff to plan workloads, and precludes premature data analysis and unco-ordinated extensions to the trial. In practice, patients may be recruited at rates differing from those predicted and interim adjustments may be agreed on.

Studies can be population based but family studies are often more effective in establishing an HLA association with disease. If the disorder is clearly inherited in families, then such studies will be essential. Of course, an analysis of the affected individuals as a disease population will also be possible. Those diseases which have no familial mode of inheritance are still worthy of family studies since family studies allow the definition of entire haplotypes, and may reveal an association between a particular haplotype and disease.

A disease population should always be limited to a single ethnic group. The frequency of HLA antigens and genes varies greatly between human populations and an ethnic mix will introduce inaccuracies. It may be the case that the association of a disease with a particular antigen or gene in one ethnic group will be with a different antigen or gene in another population. Studies of the same disease in more than one well-defined ethnic group can therefore be worthwhile.

A checklist for the design of an HLA and disease study is shown in Table 6.1.

Table 6.1   HLA and disease study criteria checklist

1. Clinical diagnostic criteria.
2. Number of patients to be included.
3. Samples types to be sent to laboratory.
4. Clinical information to be collected.
5. Study start and end times.
6. Collection of control samples.
7. Data analysis methods.
8. Conditions for publication of findings.

Controls

The establishment of an association between an HLA gene or antigen and disease depends on the comparison of patient and control data. In most studies, non-diseased or 'healthy' controls will be necessary. These are often local laboratory and hospital staff or perhaps may be drawn from blood donors. It is rarely possible to interview these people to ascertain their health status, and their co-operation in donating blood samples must be respected. It is probably unethical to question them in detail. Furthermore, blood bank donors are now a selected population, in order to avoid viral transmission, and therefore may no longer be appropriate as controls.

A useful source of control antigen frequencies can be derived from a database of cadaveric organ donors for comparison with disease groups. All of these persons were 'healthy' 24 hours prior to their death, and are divided almost equally between those suffering a fatal injury such as a road traffic accident and those suffering a brain haemorrhage. The advantage of using data from large control populations is that small disturbances in frequencies are evened out, as shown in our local study of a compilation of many different disease groups (Davidson et al., 1988). When family studies are undertaken, it is possible to use data from the family members who are not genetically related to the diseased individual(s) to compile control frequencies.

As already stated, the established differences in HLA antigen and gene frequencies over relatively small geographical areas illustrates the need for locally obtained control data. If the disease group is drawn from a specific population then control data must be obtained from that same population.

The problems of compiling control data highlight the need to determine HLA antigen and gene frequencies in well-defined 'healthy' populations. It is hoped that such data will emerge with the application of molecular methods to the definition of HLA polymorphisms. These methods place fewer restrictions on specimen transport and storage. The lesson for all laboratories is to establish local control data and to collect stored DNA, frozen viable lymphocytes and EBV-transformed cell lines for future use and reference.

Consent

It will be necessary to obtain approval for a study from the relevant ethical committee, and in all cases the patients and relatives recruited into the study should be fully informed as to the study's aims. If data are stored on computer then the constraints of the Data Protection Act must be borne in mind.

Practical aspects

Good planning will enable maximum usage of available blood samples. If several laboratories are involved in studies, often one centre can isolate samples and distribute aliquots to colleagues. Similarly, it is quite acceptable to extract DNA from the granulocytes which will sediment through the density gradient during lymphocyte preparation for serological typing.

An attempt should be made to store serum, lymphocytes (some in sterile conditions for possible EBV transformation), DNA and red blood cells to cover all possible tests. The results of one study can often suggest further work, and storage of samples avoids the need for further sample collection. Thus it is advisable to store material from patients for subsequent analysis using newly available techniques, as and when they are developed.

Some laboratories may insist for reasons of health and safety that samples are tested for virus-specific antibodies to the hepatitis viruses and to HIV before processing. This problem can be alleviated either by selecting patients who are not in high-risk groups, or by assuming that all samples are high-risk and treating them accordingly in the laboratory. Those studies which are planned in high-risk groups may require additional facilities for processing in the laboratory.

Laboratory techniques

Specimen transport and storage

Efficient ways of transporting blood samples to the laboratory should be established. For serological assays based on cytotoxicity it will be essential to minimize the delay, since non-viable lymphocytes cannot be typed reliably. Short-term transport of anticoagulated white blood should be at room temperature, but if possible lymphocytes should be isolated and transported in tissue-culture medium to preserve lymphocyte viability. For molecular biological methods, time is less important in that whole blood can be frozen at $-20°C$ and DNA extracted at a later date. Long-term storage of viable lymphocytes is achieved by cryopreservation in liquid nitrogen of cells suspended in dimethyl sulphoxide (DMSO) and fetal calf serum.

Definition of HLA antigens by serology

The microlymphocytotoxicity assay for HLA antigen typing is the established serological method in widespread use. There may be local variations to this assay, but the basic procedure is common to most laboratories (Dyer and Martin, 1991; Rodey, 1991) and involves the incubation of a pure lymphocyte population of target cells, isolated from a patient's anti-coagulated peripheral blood, with well-characterized HLA-specific human antisera. The patient's cells and the anti-HLA antibodies are incubated together for 30 minutes at 22°C to allow binding of antibodies to HLA cell surface antigens. This is followed by the addition of an excess (5 μl) of rabbit serum as a source of complement. This leads to cell killing if antibody is bound to the cell surface. Usually 2×10^3 target cells in 1 μl serum-free culture medium are incubated with 1 μl HLA-specific antiserum. In many laboratories, the assay is halted by the addition of ethylene diamine tetraacetic acid (EDTA), since complement-mediated cytotoxicity is calcium-dependent. Dead cells are identified by the addition of a vital dye that is excluded by live cells, or by two-colour fluorescence in which dead cells are stained in one colour and live cells in another. The typing plates are then 'read' by scoring each well for the percentage of cells killed. Cell lysis indicates that the cells express the HLA antigen recognized by the antiserum in an individual well.

Useful HLA typing antisera are usually obtained from multiparous women who have been sensitized against the mismatched paternal HLA antigens present on the fetus and, much less frequently, from renal transplant patients who have rejected a previous transplant. It is not an easy task to assemble a good panel of typing reagents, hence the need for collaboration between laboratories and clinical staff to ensure efficient studies of HLA-associated diseases.

Use of anti-HLA monoclonal antibodies

Monoclonal antibody technology has also been applied to tissue typing, but so far this has not been as productive as was hoped. Many anti-HLA mouse monoclonal antibodies are directed against framework determinants and do not discriminate between individual HLA types. Furthermore, some of the monoclonal antibodies that are specific for particular HLA antigens are not cytotoxic and so are not of use in the standard serological assay outlined above. Some workers have used enzyme linked immunosorbent assays (ELISA), but so far these have not found widespread use. There have also been attempts to produce monoclonal antibodies of human origin using B lymphocytes from the blood of persons with circulating HLA-specific cytotoxic antibodies, but these have also been of limited success due to the difficulty of isolating immortalized antibody-producing human B cells.

During the last few years, new techniques have been pioneered to identify HLA polymorphisms, including biochemical methods to detect polymorphisms of HLA proteins and recombinant DNA techniques to detect polymorphisms of HLA genes.

Protein chemical methods for detecting HLA antigen polymorphisms

Assays of immunoprecipitated HLA antigens after metabolic labelling in vitro with a radioactive amino acid, such as ^{35}S-methionine, have now been developed. For class I proteins, the polymorphisms are revealed by visualizing differences in isoelectric point (pI) on isoelectric focusing (IEF) gels (Yang, 1987). However, for class II molecules such an approach has been less productive, mainly because of a lack of locus-specific monoclonal antibodies for immunoprecipitation: usually more than one class II chain is bound by available monoclonal antibodies. Furthermore, both the α and the β chains of DQ and DP molecules are polymorphic, in contrast to class I antigens where only the heavy chain is polymorphic. The class I light chain, β2 microglobulin, which is encoded outside the MHC on chromosome 15, is not polymorphic, as discussed in Chapter 1.

One approach to the resolution of class II polymorphism by biochemical techniques has been to use two-dimensional gels. Immunoprecipitates are first run into an SDS gel, leading to separation by molecular weight. The gels are then run in a second dimension, at 90 degrees to the first, using a pH gradient to reveal pI differences (IEF). Unfortunately, interpretation of the resulting autoradiographs is not straightforward and quantification is not possible (Knowles, 1989).

Recombinant DNA techniques for detecting HLA gene polymorphisms

By contrast to protein-based techniques, the development of recombinant DNA technology has led to substantial progress in the definition of class II polymorphisms. Initially, restriction fragment length polymorphism (RFLP) analysis of HLA-DR and DQ genes was used (Bidwell and Bignon, 1991). However, RFLP typing adds relatively little to the information that can be acquired using conventional serological techniques.

With the recent definition of HLA class II gene sequences, several groups have developed typing systems based on the amplification of DNA using the polymerase chain reaction (PCR). Several techniques are currently employed routinely. The presence of a particular allele can be detected by the ability to generate a PCR product using sequence-specific primers (SSPs) (Olerup and Zetterquist, 1992). Alternatively, 'universal' primers may be used to amplify all alleles of a single HLA class II gene and the product can then be analysed by one of several techniques to define the allele. The PCR product may be subjected to gel electrophoresis, blotted on to a nylon membrane and probed with labelled allele- or sequence-specific oligonucleotides (ASOs or SSOs) (Fernandez-Vina et al., 1991). Alternatively, PCR products may be captured on plates coated with a specific ASO or SSO and the presence of bound product may be detected colorimetrically using a universal enzyme-linked oligonucleotide. Yet another approach has been to combine PCR amplification with restriction enzyme digestion, which also avoids the use of radioactive probes; there are now several novel approaches in this area (Uryu et al., 1990). The development of non-radioactive probes, by labelling with molecules such as digoxigenin (DIG), have speeded up many of these methods (Nevinny-Stickel et al., 1991). These are very powerful approaches, and are capable of resolving the differences between many subtypes of serologically defined specificities that could previously only be routinely distinguished using cellular typing, such as the 12 subtypes of HLA-DR4.

The ultimate approach to HLA typing is to sequence the coding regions of MHC genes and methods to do this rapidly on a large number of individuals, using PCR-amplified DNA, are now appearing (Gyllensten and Erlich, 1988).

During the past few years, a large number of genes have been located within the MHC which code for non-cell surface molecules. Several of these genes have been shown to be polymorphic. These are detailed in Chapter 9. Polymorphisms of these genes can be defined using one or more of the above techniques and may have direct relevance to disease associations because of the influence of their gene products on the immune response. Indeed, given their very close linkage to class I and class II genes, it is possible that these non-HLA genes may prove to be the true susceptibility genes in some of the 'so-called' HLA-associated diseases.

Other methods, such as long-range mapping by pulsed-field gel electrophoresis (PFGE) using restriction endonucleases that cleave DNA only rarely have enabled the detection of deletions within the MHC. One such example, occurring in the class III region, leads to 21-hydroxylase deficiency and congenital adrenal hyperplasia (Collier et al., 1989). Recently, techniques to identify size differences between MHC haplotypes due to deletions or duplications have been developed (Kendall et al., 1991) which also might have relevance to disease associations (Cross et al., 1991; Jongeneel et al., 1991).

Use of cell lines

With the development of these new techniques there is a diminishing need to perform functional cellular assays in the analysis of HLA polymorphism. However, it is wise to immortalize patient samples by creation of cell lines from B lymphocytes by infection with the Epstein–Barr virus (Neitzel, 1986). This guarantees unlimited supplies of viable cells which will also yield DNA for molecular biological assays.

Collection of clinical data and data handling

It is important to establish a thorough and efficient protocol for recording of relevant clinical information. Relevant items include family history and a checklist of known HLA-associated diseases, as well as the details specific to the disease under study.

Both clinical data and laboratory data should be stored on computer. This will aid efficient storage of data for subsequent retrieval and analysis. There are many database software packages commercially available, but choice of a popular package will facilitate sharing of data with other workers. At the outset, it should be established which study collaborators will have access to the data. It is often best to deny all access until the study is completed!

Nomenclature

Usually, well-defined diseases will have accepted diagnostic criteria which are accompanied by a recognized nomenclature; to avoid confusion this should always be used. If such a nomenclature is not available, the launching of an HLA and disease study may provide an opportunity to propose a standard. With regard to HLA nomenclature, one reason why our knowledge of the MHC has grown so rapidly has been the remarkable international collaboration through the WHO HLA Nomenclature Committee. Updates to the WHO HLA nomenclature are published following every HLA International Workshop. Reports are found in histocompatibility and immunogenetics journals. Recently, with the rapid developments resulting from molecular biology techniques, there have been interim reports following international conferences and again these updates are widely published. Familiarization with current HLA nomenclature at the outset of a disease study will simplify data presentation for publication purposes when the study is concluded. The current system of nomenclature is explained in Chapter 2.

Quality assurance

There are several steps which can be taken to monitor and guarantee the quality of laboratory data in a study. A check of data is possible if both serological and molecular typing is performed; a good correlation between antigen (serology) and gene (molecular) frequencies should be found. Studies in which there are discrepancies between the frequency of an antigen and the gene that encodes it are invalid due to poor laboratory technique.

The incidence of persons typed as 'apparent homozygotes', that is having only one antigen at a given locus, is a good indicator of the efficiency and quality of serological methods, since this figure should be very similar in published and control data. This is discussed further below.

Statistical methods

Consideration of some fundamental statistical principles is necessary in the design and the interpretation of HLA and disease studies. These principles will influence the size of the study, the choice of a population-based or a family study, and the selection of controls. The key statistical concepts are outlined here, but reference may need to be made to a fuller statistical text for a more detailed discussion.

Population studies

If individuals with different HLA antigens have varying risks of disease, then a difference should be seen in the distribution of HLA types between patients and healthy controls. The objective of population (association) studies is then to compare the frequencies of specific HLA antigens in a series of patients with those seen in a series of controls. If one or more of the antigens are significantly increased in frequency in cases over controls then there is said to be an association between the disease and HLA. However, although it is tempting to assume that any such association represents an increased risk of disease to carriers of that HLA antigen, other explanations should be considered (see 'The biological interpretation of an association between an antigen and the disease' below).

To make this comparison meaningful, the controls must be as similar to the cases as possible except, of course, in their disease state. Since antigen frequencies vary with ethnicity and geographical region, these factors must be considered when deciding how to collect a series of controls (as discussed above). Failure to provide such compatibility of patients and controls might produce spurious evidence of an association. For instance, if controls came from a different ethnic background from that of the patients and differences were detected in HLA antigen frequencies between these two ethnic groups (unrelated to the disease), then, in the context of a disease study, these differences would be interpreted incorrectly as an association between the disease and HLA.

Identifying associations between antigens and disease

Table 6.2 shows a fictitious study in which 96 patients with a defined condition were typed for the DR locus. A total of 504 individuals from the same racial group were typed as controls. Each line of the table shows the number of patients or controls that typed positively for one of the antigens. Although the absolute numbers in the table are not easily interpreted, examination of the percentages show that DR2 is increased in frequency among the cases while all the other antigens (except DR1) are reduced in frequency when compared to the controls. (The frequency of DR1 is almost the same in both groups.) The main question arising from these data is whether or not there is a statistically significant association between this disease and the presence of DR2. The difference between 29.8% and 75.0% is striking. However, until statistically analysed, it remains possible that this apparent difference arose by chance. Not all changes in frequency are meaningful. Obviously, if DR2 is positively associated with disease and there are no other associations (positive or negative), there will be a compensatory decrease in the frequency of other DR allotypes.

To decide whether the discrepancy in the frequency of DR2 in the two groups is statistically significant, the summary given in Table 6.3 is constructed. This table is termed a '2 × 2 contingency table'. Cases and controls are documented in separate

Table 6.2 Example of data from population study of HLA and disease association

Antigen	Controls (n = 504)		Patients (n = 96)	
	Number positive	% positive	Number positive	% positive
DR1	105	20.8	21	21.9
DR2	150	29.8	74	75.0
DR3	150	29.8	11	11.5
DR4	172	34.2	29	30.2
DR6	107	21.2	17	18.0
DR7	122	24.2	12	12.5
DR8	16	3.4	1	1.0
DR9	8	1.7	1	1.0
DR10	5	1.0	0	0
DR11	46	9.1	6	6.3
DR12	5	1.0	0	0

Table 6.3 2 × 2 contingency table summarizing for DR2 data in Table 6.2

	DR2$^+$ individuals	DR2$^-$ individuals	Totals
Patients	74	22	96
Controls	150	354	504
Totals	224	376	600

rows of the table, the number positive for DR2 is shown in the first column, and the number negative for DR2 is shown in the second column. The row sum for the first row of the table must equal the number of cases studied while the second row must sum to the number of controls in the series.

The standard statistical approach to the question of significance is to estimate the probability that this pattern of frequencies of antigen-positive and -negative cases and antigen-positive and -negative controls could have arisen by chance alone. If the probability of making these observations was very low then we may conclude that it did not arise by chance and there really is some association between DR2 and this disease.

How do we estimate the probability of obtaining these data by chance? If we assume there is no association (which is the 'null hypothesis'), being a case or a control is independent of the presence or absence of the antigen. How far do the observed data differ from what would be expected? Of the total 600 individuals examined, 224 were DR2$^+$. In the absence of an association, of the 96 patients, 35.84 [i.e. (224/600) × 96] would be expected to be DR2$^+$ and the remaining 60.16 would be expected to be DR2$^-$. (Fractions of people, ludicrous in reality, do have statistical meaning, in the same way that one speaks of an average family having 2.4 children.) The frequencies expected if the null hypothesis is correct can be calculated in a similar way for the controls. We use these observed (O) and expected (E) data to calculate a test statistic (approximating to the chi-square statistic) to estimate the significance of this apparent association. This statistic is calculated using the formula:

$$\Sigma\,(O-E)^2/E \qquad (6.1)$$

The Greek letter sigma indicates the sum of all values for $(O-E)^2/E$. The test statistic in the 2 × 2 contingency table for these data is therefore the sum of the four values

Table 6.4 Calculation of test statistic to apply the chi-square test to the data displayed in Table 6.3

	DR2$^+$ individuals				
	Observed (O)	Expected (E)	$O-E$	$(O-E)^2$	$(O-E)^2/E$
Patients	74	(224/600) × 96 = 35.84	74 − 35.84 = 38.16	1456.18	40.63
Controls	150	(224/600) × 504 = 188.16	150 − 188.16 = −38.16	1456.18	7.74

	DR2$^-$ individuals				
	Observed (O)	Expected (E)	$O-E$	$(O-E)^2$	$(O-E)^2/E$
Patients	22	(376/600) × 96 = 60.16	22 − 60.16 = −38.16	1456.18	24.21
Controls	354	(376/600) × 504 = 315.84	354 − 315.84 = 38.16	1456.18	4.61

$\Sigma(O-E)^2/E = 40.63 + 7.74 + 24.21 + 4.61 = 77.19$

calculated for $(O-E)^2/E$, for these data, the sum of 40.63, 7.74, 24.21 and 4.61, i.e. 77.19. (The calculation is summarized in Table 6.4). There is further discussion of how the chi-square test works in the appendix.

Large values of the test statistic imply that the observed data have not arisen by chance. To determine whether a test statistic is 'large', one consults tables of the chi-square distribution. To do so, it is necessary to know the number of 'degrees of freedom' and the level of statistical significance required. (The concept of 'degrees of freedom' is discussed further in the appendix.) For each number of degrees of freedom, the chi-square distribution is different. This can be represented graphically, and some examples are provided in the appendix (Appendix, Figure 6.A8). If the area under such a graph is calculated it is possible to plot a value for χ^2 which divides the lower 95% of the area from the top 5%. This means that if the value of the calculated test statistic is greater than that value of χ^2, then there is only a 5% probability that this value came from that distribution, or $P < 0.05$. The value chosen for P, defines the level of statistical significance being employed. If the test statistic does give such a large value, this means that it is so unlikely that this test statistic comes from this chi-square distribution, that you do not believe the initial (null) hypothesis, and you may conclude, with statistical justification, that there is an association between your HLA antigen and this disease.

Table 6.5 provides an extract from a table of the chi-square distribution. In this, the values of χ^2 for three levels of statistical significance are given for the chi-square distribution for various degrees of freedom. In the case of the 2×2 contingency table, there is one degree of freedom. The first line of Table 6.5 gives values of χ^2 for the

Table 6.5 Sample of tabulated values of chi-square distribution for various degrees of freedom

Degrees of freedom	$P = 0.05$	$P = 0.01$	$P = 0.001$
1	3.841	6.635	10.827
2	5.991	9.210	13.815
3	7.815	11.345	16.266
4	9.488	13.277	18.467
5	11.070	15.086	20.515
6	12.592	16.812	22.457
7	14.067	18.475	24.322
8	15.507	20.090	26.125
9	16.919	21.666	27.877
10	18.307	23.209	29.588
11	19.675	24.725	31.264
12	21.026	26.217	32.909
13	22.362	27.688	34.528
14	23.685	29.141	36.123
15	24.996	30.578	37.697
16	26.296	32.000	39.252
17	27.587	33.409	40.790
18	28.869	34.805	42.312
19	30.144	36.191	43.820
20	31.410	37.566	45.315
30	43.773	50.892	59.703
40	55.759	63.691	73.402
50	67.505	76.154	86.661
60	79.082	88.379	99.607

distribution of chi-square with one degree of freedom. For a significance level of 0.05 (i.e. $P < 0.05$) the value of the test statistic must be at least 3.84 and for a significance level of 0.01, at least 6.64. In the case of these example data, the test statistic is 77.19, far larger than either of these minimum values, indeed larger than the minimum value for significance at the 0.001 level, i.e. there is less than 0.1% likelihood that these data could have occurred by chance. Accordingly, we say that the null hypothesis falls and we may conclude that this sample demonstrates that there is a statistically highly significant association between the antigen and the disease. It is possible to calculate a value of χ^2 at any given value of P. In essence, you would be calculating the value of χ^2 above which a proportion P of the area under the relevant chi-square distribution occurred (Appendix, Figures 6.A7 and 6.A8). In practice, one is most interested in P values of 0.05, 0.01 and 0.001, and these are tabulated in Table 6.5.

The chi-squared distribution is only an approximation to the true distribution appropriate for the test statistic, $\Sigma(O-E)^2/E$. There are two sources of error if it is applied inappropriately. Firstly, it cannot be applied to small samples. A rule of thumb which is widely accepted is that 80% of *expected* frequencies (E) must exceed five and none must be less than one (Bland, 1987). However, the exact limits of size for the chi-square test remains an area of debate among statisticians. For a 2×2 contingency table, this means, in practice, that all four values of E must exceed five.

The second problem arises from the fact that we are using the 'continuous' chi square distribution to deal with a 'discrete' distribution. This discrete distribution can be made to fit more closely to the continuous chi-square distribution by introducing Yates' continuity correction, which is how the statistic is often tabulated. (This is discussed further in the appendix.) However, Yates' correction may result in an over-conservative test and the consequent missing of a significant association. Statisticians are divided on whether or not it should be used (Bland, 1987; Daniel, 1987). The correction, strictly, is not necessary for large sample sizes, but it only meaningfully affects the result when the sample size is small.

If the expected frequencies are too small to use the chi-square test, an alternative statistic, generated by Fisher's exact test, is used. A description of the principle of this test is included in the appendix. Many statistical software programs for 2×2 tables perform this calculation routinely and warn when Fisher's exact test must be considered because the sample sizes are not appropriate for the chi-square test.

There are additional features that complicate the analysis of disease associations with HLA antigens. Due to the extreme polymorphism of the HLA system, most of the phenotypes observed will be seen in only a small proportion of cases and controls. It is possible to include multiple alleles in the same comparison. However, since there is a risk of generating false-positive results, a correction factor for the number of tests must be included. This will be discussed further below.

An additional complication arises because of the presence of two or more copies of all loci in each individual. A case or control who is typed positive for only a single antigen by serology may either carry two copies of the same allele, or he may carry one copy of the allele in question and a second allele encoding an antigen for which no antisera are available. The lack of serological definition can only be removed if family information is available. In this case, typing family members can elucidate the presence of a 'blank' allele. If blank alleles are rare, then such approaches are not usually necessary and homozygosity can be assumed. When the percentages of individuals with each antigen are added together and the total subtracted from 200%

Table 6.6 Estimation of homozygosity from observed antigen frequencies in the absence of a significant prevalence of serologically 'blank' alleles

Antigen	Controls ($n = 504$) % positive	Patients ($n = 96$) % positive
DR1	20.8	21.9
DR2	29.8	75.0
DR3	29.8	11.5
DR4	34.2	30.2
DR6	21.2	18.0
DR7	24.2	12.5
DR8	3.4	1.0
DR9	1.7	1.0
DR10	1.0	0
DR11	9.1	6.3
DR12	1.0	0
Total	176.2	178.1
Apparent homozygotes	$200 - 176.2 = 23.8$	$200 - 178.1 = 21.9$

(i.e. two copies of each locus per person), the remaining figure represents the proportion of 'apparent homozygotes'. Table 6.6 illustrates such a situation. Such issues will not in general arise when DNA analysis of the HLA system is performed instead of serological analysis.

Measuring the strength of the association

If there is evidence of a significant association, then a method for indicating the strength of the association is required. The usual measure of the strength of an association is the risk of disease among those positive for the antigen compared to those without the antigen, as suggested initially by Woolf (1955). A strong association is one in which the risk among carriers is either much larger or much smaller than the risk to non-carriers. Using the nomenclature of Table 6.7, if the disease is rare, then the ratio of these risks can be estimated by ad/bc. This ratio for the estimation of relative risk can be derived as follows. The prevalence of the disease in individuals positive for the antigen can be expressed as $(a/c) \times k$ and the prevalence of disease in antigen-negative individuals as $(b/d) \times k$. We have to introduce an unknown constant (k) because we have no information about the absolute prevalence of the disease. However, the same constant is applied to both a/c and b/d. The 'relative incidence' or 'relative risk' (RR) can be calculated using the formula:

$$\text{RR} = \frac{(a/c) \times k}{(b/d) \times k} = \frac{a/c}{b/d} = \frac{ad}{bc} \tag{6.2}$$

A relative risk close to 1.0 implies that those carrying the antigen have no increased risk of disease, i.e. there is no association between the antigen and disease expression. A relative risk greater than 1.0 implies that those carrying the antigen are at increased risk of disease (a positive association), while a relative risk less than 1.0 implies those carrying the antigen are at lower risk of expressing the disease than those not carrying the antigen (a negative association). The further the number deviates from 1, the stronger the association.

106   P. Dyer and A. Warrens

Table 6.7   Symbolic representation of 2 × 2 contingency table to illustrate the calculation of relative risk

	Number of individuals	
	Positive for the antigen	Negative for the antigen
Patients	a	b
Controls	c	d

The statistical interpretation of an association between an antigen and the disease

How do we evaluate the results of a particular study? Clearly a relative risk of 3.0 would be much more exciting if it were obtained with a sample of 1000 patients and controls than if achieved with a sample size of 20 in each group. The relative risk obtained from the smaller sample size could simply be due to chance because an unusual sample could produce this inflated estimate even if there were really no association; such an explanation would be much less plausible for the larger sample size. The interpretation then depends upon the sample size and is measured by the statistical significance.

With the 2 × 2 contingency table, we used the chi-square test to measure how far each of the observed frequencies deviate from an expected value ('expected' if all values were taken from the same population). The statistical significance of a relative risk can similarly be calculated using the chi-square distribution, by making an estimate of the deviation of each of the figures represented by a, b, c and d in the formula above. This is discussed further in the appendix.

Using the data in Table 6.8 as an example, the estimated relative risk for the whole population for the association between DR3 and the disease is 4.7 (= 65 × 440/151 × 40). This means that there is evidence suggestive of a strong positive association between the antigen and the disease. Using the formula presented in the appendix, these data generate a test statistic for the chi-square test of 48.60, much greater than 3.84, which makes this RR highly statistically significant.

Table 6.8   Example of 2 × 2 contingency table to illustrate the calculation of relative risk

	Number of individuals	
	DR3$^+$	DR3$^-$
Patients ($n=105$)	65	40
Controls ($n=591$)	151	440

For small values of a, b, c or d, Haldane has introduced a modification of the formula to calculate RR (Haldane, 1956). This is discussed further in the appendix.

We have discussed the application of statistical tests to the simple 2 × 2 contingency table and the evaluation of relative risk. The application of statistical analysis becomes much more involved with more complex data, as is illustrated in the following example.

Let us postulate a disease in whose aetiology we believe HLA may be involved. We conduct an association study in the standard way. In particular, we examine the association between the disease and each of the alleles of this particular HLA locus. On performing a chi-square test, we find that several antigens show evidence of an association. Before becoming too enthusiastic about the results, we should re-examine the meaning of the phrase 'statistical significance'. The significance level we have calculated for each antigen is the probability that a result as extreme as this would occur if there truly were no association. A significance level of 0.05 means that one out of 20 analyses conducted when there is really no association, would produce a result as extreme as this by chance, i.e. would erroneously suggest an association. Put another way, even if there is no relationship between HLA and this disease, were we to examine 20 antigens using a significance level of 0.05 we could expect one of the antigens to show evidence of an association by having a chi-square test statistic with a value of at least 3.84.

How then do we decide on the importance of the results of a particular study? Since the analysis of each antigen that is typed for can spuriously produce evidence of an association, the usual approach is to calculate the significance level of each test and to multiply that result by the number of statistical tests performed. This 'corrected' significance level is then reported as the statistical significance of the test. For instance, if one particular HLA locus is examined, then one statistical test is performed for each antigen that was typed, so the number of statistical tests is equal to the number of antigens. For instance, if we define 20 HLA-DR types in a particular study, and the significance level of one of the DR types is 0.001, then the reported value for that analysis should be modified to 0.02 (=20 × 0.001). This approach is

Table 6.9 Data from original study (Schlosstein et al., 1973) demonstrating association of HLA-B27 with ankylosing spondylitis. Used here to illustrate application of Bonferoni correction factor (see text for full discussion)

Antigen	Cases of ankylosing spondylitis (%) ($n = 40$)	Controls (%) ($n = 906$)
A1	10	27
A2	60	48
A3	18	24
A9	30	22
A10	8	11
A11	10	12
A28	18	12
A29	10	7
A30	15	10
A32	13	8
B51	5	11
B7	3[a]	25
B8	15	21
B44	18	24
B13	3	4
B35	18	22
B40	18	14
B14	5	7
B15	8	8
B17	5	8
B18	5	9
B21	3	5
B22	3	5
B27	88[b]	8

[a] Chi-square = 9.32 ($P < 0.05$ when multiplied by 24).
[b] Chi-square = 236.41 ($P < 0.0001$ when multiplied by 24, number of specificities tested.).

called the Bonferoni correction [see Dunn (1961) for a detailed discussion, or a statistics textbook for a more general presentation]. If the corrected significance level is still less than 0.05 then this is taken as an indication of a genuine association between that antigen and the disease. Any antigen for which the corrected value is greater than 0.05 would not be considered to be associated with the disease.

Table 6.9 reproduces one of the original studies that described the association between ankylosing spondylitis (AS) and HLA-B27 (Schlosstein et al., 1973). Initial inspection suggests a strong association, with a much larger incidence of B27 in the AS group than the controls. Application of the Bonferoni correction factor confirms the positive association with B27 and a much weaker negative one with B7.

One way to circumvent problems caused by applying Bonferoni's correction factor is to focus the study design on a very specific question. Suppose a colleague has published a study reporting evidence of an association of the disease in question with a specific HLA antigen. We are interested in confirming this association, so we study a group of patients with the same disease and examine in particular, the association with that antigen, using the statistical method previously described. The advantage of this kind of confirmatory study is that, because of information from the previous study, attention can be focused on a single HLA antigen, thus greatly reducing the correction factor. The earlier study should also provide us with an estimate of the strength of the association. On the basis of that estimate, and allowing for a margin of error, it should be possible to estimate the size of sample required to perform a study with adequate statistical power to detect an association of similar magnitude. This is preferable to finding after the study is completed that the statistical analysis does not achieve significance, and then attempting to achieve significance by collecting more samples.

The biological interpretation of an association between an antigen and a disease

The identification of a statistical association between an antigen and a disease could indicate one of several underlying biological phenomena. The first is that the HLA antigen itself is responsible for conferring susceptibility to disease. However, an alternative explanation is that there is a disease locus which is within the HLA region of the chromosome but is not itself part of the HLA system. In this case, there would be a 'linkage disequilibrium' between the disease locus and one or more of the HLA loci, as the result of the physical proximity of the genes and the recency of the mutation causing susceptibility in the disease gene. As a result, a disproportionate percentage of patients bear the haplotype that existed in the patient who suffered the original mutation. In such a setting, there may well be associations with a number of HLA loci because of the linkage disequilibrium between the HLA loci themselves. In theory, the strength of each association could be used to identify the closest HLA locus, but in practice the ability to make such interpretations is limited (see, for an example, Thomson and Bodmer, 1977).

Two haplotype effects can also be observed, as evidenced by disease associations with more than one HLA antigen or allele. One of the best examples of a two haplotype effect is the association of HLA-DR3 and -DR4 with insulin-dependent diabetes mellitus (IDDM). In this case, although there is a significant association between both DR3 and DR4, as individual antigens, with IDDM, there is actually a stronger association with heterozygosity for DR3 and DR4. The possible mechanisms underlying two such haplotype effects are discussed in Chapter 7.

Family studies

If a disease-causing gene is not itself an HLA gene, but is located close to an HLA molecule-encoding gene, then a family study is usually the most convenient and often the only way to identify the association. The method relies upon linkage between genes, i.e. the tendency for both genes to segregate together in families [see Cavalli-Sforza and Bodmer (1971) for more details of linkage]. If the linkage is very tight so that the disease gene essentially always segregates with HLA, and the disease causing mutation has occurred recently enough, then it may be possible to detect the association using a population-based method (as described above). The conditions under which such an association could be identified are relatively restrictive and in their absence, a family study will usually be required to identify the linkage.

Family studies are based on the following observations. Suppose a family has two children. Both parents are typed: the father's haplotypes are A and B and the mother's, C and D. There are four possible haplotype pairings for each child (AC, AD, BC and BD), making 16 possible combinations of HLA types for the two children (see Table 6.10). A, B, C and D could represent the typing results either from a single or multiple HLA loci. In the latter case, they are termed 'haplotypes'. The 16 possibilities can be classified usefully to one of three categories depending on the number of haplotypes that the two sibs share. If the two sibs are identical at both HLA loci (combinations 1, 6, 11 and 16 in Table 6.10), then they are said to share two haplotypes (i.e. the same haplotype from each parent), while two sibs who are entirely discordant for the HLA alleles inherited from the parents (combinations 4, 7, 10 and 13) are said to share zero haplotypes. The other possibility is that the sibs share exactly one set of alleles, in which case the sibs have inherited the same haplotype from one parent and different haplotypes from the other parent. The haplotypes A, B, C and D will be different in different families but for each family the typing results are reduced to the number of shared haplotypes among the children.

Table 6.10 Possible combinations of parental haplotypes in two siblings

Combination	Child 1	Child 2	Combination	Child 1	Child 2
1	AC	AC	9	AC	BC
2	AD	AC	10	AD	BC
3	BC	AC	11	BC	BC
4	BD	AC	12	BD	BC
5	AC	AD	13	AC	BD
6	AD	AD	14	AD	BD
7	BC	AD	15	BC	BD
8	BD	AD	16	BD	BD

The method of identifying disease-linked genes using family studies was originally suggested by Penrose (1935) who realized that the sharing of haplotypes would be modified if the typed locus was genetically linked to a disease-causing gene. In particular, sibs affected with the same disease should show more sharing of parental haplotypes than would be predicted by chance. To identify a linkage, the observed pattern of haplotype sharing among sibs must be compared with the distribution of haplotypes that would occur if the disease gene and the typed gene were unlinked to each other. In the latter case, the 16 possibilities of Table 6.10 would be equally likely,

Table 6.11   Results of sibling-pair study of Ebers et al. (1982)

Haplotypes shared	Expected	Observed
2	10	12
1	20	18
0	10	10

so that the probability that the sibs share two haplotypes is 0.25, one haplotype is 0.5 and zero haplotypes is 0.25. Any evidence of excess sharing over this distribution is consistent with linkage. For instance, in Table 6.11, the result of a study by Ebers et al. (1982) of sibs with multiple sclerosis is shown. In 40 sib-pairs drawn from 36 families, the haplotype sharing among two affected siblings was identified. Twelve shared two haplotypes, 18 shared one haplotype and ten shared no haplotypes. This can be compared with the expected result of ten pairs sharing two haplotypes, 20 pairs sharing one haplotype and ten sharing no haplotypes. There is therefore only a trivial increase in HLA sharing among the MS siblings. Again the observed and expected sharing can be compared using a chi-square test. In this case, the test statistic is not significant showing that there is no evidence of excess of HLA sharing among the MS siblings. A value of 5.99 or greater would have given evidence at a significance level of 0.05 (given that there are two degrees of freedom – see Table 6.5) and would be interpreted as evidence of linkage, provided that the observed distribution of shared haplotypes is in the direction of increased haplotypes over the expected. More detailed discussions of this method can be found in Green and Woodrow (1977), Day and Simons (1976), and Fishman et al. (1978).

The statistical method described above is simplistic in that it does not take into account any features of the disease transmission in families. Such information is often not well known, in which case this method is appropriate. However, if there is further information, such as an indication as to whether the disease is inherited as an autosomal dominant or a recessive trait, then this can be incorporated and utilized to produce a more powerful test of linkage. One approach to this is the application of the method of log odds ratios or 'lod scores'. This is discussed further in the appendix and further details of and references to such methods can be found in Cavalli-Sforza and Bodmer (1971) and Ott (1991).

Data communication

Publication of results

In the past there have been many publications of data from HLA and disease studies, and most major diseases have been examined. It is now unusual to publish studies based on serological methods alone, since molecular genetic techniques provide much more information. If there has been a bias in past publications it has been to withhold the reporting of negative data. Such data are important, if only to prevent unnecessary studies by other workers.

Scientific journals in the immunogenetics field are the usual location for the publication of study results but for novel findings major clinical journals which are widely read may publish data. It is most important that new gene sequence data from a study is entered into one of the accepted registries for the use and benefit of other workers. In some journals, registration is a condition of publication of the data.

Clinical value of defining HLA and disease associations

The value of defining associations between HLA antigens and disease is largely related to the insight that such observations provide into possible mechanisms of disease pathogenesis. Clearly most, if not all, HLA-associated diseases are polygenic. When other susceptibility genes are defined, knowledge of HLA susceptibility factors may also help to define an "at risk" population for any preventive measures that become applicable. In the short term, there is little justification for HLA typing of individual patients as a service investigation because the associations are incomplete, the relative risks are low and there are few, if any, implications for patient management. The frequency of disease-associated HLA antigens in healthy persons is usually sufficient to deny meaningful interpretation of results from a single patient. One of the few possible exceptions to this rule is ankylosing spondylitis. It is not uncommon for routine HLA testing laboratories to provide a service for HLA-B27 typing to aid in the diagnosis of this disease, largely because it has such a high relative risk (RR > 80).

Conclusion

This is a particularly exciting time in the field of HLA and disease studies, as stated at the start of this chapter. In addition to the points made earlier, many autoimmune, HLA-associated diseases are being dissected in vitro by the careful definition of the autoantigens, the production of autoantigen-specific T-cell clones, and the characterization of the T-cell receptors involved in autoreactivity. These areas of progress mean that it will soon be possible to ascribe mechanisms to some of the well-defined HLA and disease associations. Furthermore, the discovery of multiple additional genes within the HLA region, many with as yet unknown functions, opens up new possibilities to account for some HLA and disease associations. The final ingredient that makes this such a promising period for understanding the contributions of the HLA region to genetic susceptibility to disease is the rapid advances in the techniques available for the definition of polymorphism. Technology has changed radically during the past few years, and undoubtedly is not yet terminally differentiated!

Although most of the major chronic immunologically mediated diseases have been the subject of HLA studies, this should not in any way deter current investigators from designing a study that will capitalize on one or more of these recent advances.

References

Bidwell, J.L. and Bignon, J.D. (1991). DNA-RFLP methods and interpretation scheme for HLA-DR and DQ typing. *Eur. J. Immunogenet.* **18**: 5–22.

Bjorkman, P.J., Saper, M.A., Samraoui, B., Bennett, W.S., Strominger, J.L. and Wiley, D.C. (1987). Structure of the human Class I histocompatibility antigen, HLA-A2. *Nature* **329**: 506–512.

Bland, M. (1987). *An Introduction to Medical Statistics.* Oxford University Press, Oxford.

Brewerton, D.A., Caffrey, M., Hart, F.D., James, D.C.O., Nicholls, A. and Sturrock, R.D. (1973). Ankylosing spondylitis and HL-A27. *Lancet* **i**: 904–907.

Cavalli-Sforza, L.L. and Bodmer, W.F. (1971). *The Genetics of Human Populations.* W.H. Freeman and Company, San Francisco.

Collier, S., Sinnott, P.J., Dyer, P.A., Price, D.A., Harris, R. and Strachan, T. (1989). Pulsed field gel electrophoresis identifies a high degree of variability in the number of tandem 21-hydroxylase and complement C4 gene repeats in 21-hydroxylase deficiency haplotypes. *EMBO J.* **8**: 1393–1402.

Cross, S.J., Tonks, S., Trowsdale, J. and Campbell, R.D. (1991). Novel detection of restriction fragment length polymorphisms in the human major histocompatibility complex. *Immunogenetics* **34**: 376–384.

Daniel, W.W. (1987). *Biostatistics: A Foundation for Analysis in the Health Sciences.* John Wiley, New York, pp. 552–553.

Davidson, J.A., Kippax, R.L. and Dyer, P.A. (1988). A study of HLA-A, B, DR and Bf bearing haplotypes derived from 304 families resident in the north west of England. *J. Immunogenet.* **15**: 227–237.

Day, N.E. and Simons, M.J. (1976). Disease susceptibility genes – their identification by multiple case family studies. *Tissue Antigens* **8**: 109–119.

Dunn, O.J. (1961). Multiple comparisons among means. *Am. J. Stat. Assoc.* **56**: 52–64.

Dyer, P.A. and Martin, S. (1991). Techniques used to define human MHC antigens: serology. *Immunol. Lett.* **29**: 15–22.

Ebers, G.C., Paty, D.W., Stiller, C.R., Nelson, R.F., Seland, T.P. and Larsen, B. (1982). HLA typing in multiple sclerosis sibling pairs. *Lancet* **ii**: 88–90.

Fernandez-Vina, M.A., Gao, X., Moraes, M.E., Moraes, J.R., Salatiel, I., Miller, S., Tsai, J., Sun, Y., An, J., Layrisse, Z., Gazit, E., Brautbar, C. and Stastny, P. (1991). Alleles at four HLA class II loci determined by oligonucleotide hybridization and their associations in five ethnic groups. *Immunogenetics* **34**: 299–312.

Fishman, P.M., Suarez, B., Hodge, S.E. and Reich, T. (1978). A robust method for the detection of linkage in familial disease. *Am. J. Hum. Genet.* **30**: 308–321.

Green, J.R. and Woodrow, J.C. (1977). Sibling method for detecting HLA-linked genes in disease. *Tissue Antigens* **9**: 31–35.

Gyllensten, U.B. and Erlich, H.A. (1988). Generation of single stranded DNA by the polymerase chain reaction and its application to direct sequencing of the HLA-DQA locus. *Proc. Natl Acad. Sci. USA* **85**: 7652–7656.

Haldane, J.B.S. (1956). The estimation and significance of the logarithm of a ratio of frequencies. *Ann. Hum. Genet.* **20**: 309–311.

Jongeneel, C.V., Briant, L., Udalova, I.A., Sevin, A., Nedospasov, S.A. and Cambon-Thomsen, A. (1991). Extensive genetic polymorphism in the human tumour necrosis factor region and relation to extended HLA haplotypes. *Proc. Natl Acad. Sci. USA* **88**: 9717–9721.

Kendall, E., Todd, J.A. and Campbell, R.D. (1991). Molecular analysis of the MHC class II region in DR4, DR7 and DR9 haplotypes. *Immunogenetics* **34**: 349–357.

Knowles, R.W. (1989). Structural polymorphism of the HLA class II α and β chains: summary of the 10th Workshop 2-D gel analysis. In *Immunobiology of HLA*, Vol. 1 (ed. B. Dupont), pp. 365–380, Springer-Verlag, New York.

Neitzel, H. (1986). A routine method for the establishment of permanent growing lymphoblastoid cell lines. *Hum. Genet.* **73**: 320–326.

Nevinny-Stickel, G., Hinzpeter, M., Andreas, A. and Albert, E.D. (1991). Non-radioactive oligotyping for HLA-DR1-DRw10 using polymerase chain reaction, digoxigenin-labelled oligonucleotides and chemiluminescence detection. *Eur. J. Immunogenet.* **18**: 323–332.

Olerup, O. and Zetterquist, H. (1992). HLA-DR typing by PCR amplification with sequence-specific primers (PCR-SSP) in 2 hours: an alternative to serological DR typing in clinical practice including donor-recipient matching in cadaveric transplantation. *Tissue Antigens* **39**: 225–235.

Ott, J. (1991). *Analysis of Human Genetic Linkage*. The Johns Hopkins University Press, Baltimore.

Penrose, L.S. (1935). The detection of autosomal linkage in data which consists of pairs of brothers and sisters of unspecified parentage. *Ann. Eugenics* **6**: 133–138.

Rodey, G.E. (1991). *HLA Beyond Tears*. De Novo, Atlanta, GA.

Schlosstein, L., Terasaki, P.I., Bluestone, R. and Pearson, G.M. (1973). High association of an HL-A antigen, w27, with ankylosing spondylitis. *N. Engl. J. Med.* **288**: 704–706.

Thomson, G. and Bodmer, W. (1977). The genetic analysis of HLA and disease associations. In *HLA and Disease* (eds J. Dausset and A. Svejgaard), pp. 84–93, Munksgaard, Copenhagen.

Tiwari, J.L. and Terasaki, P.I. (1985). *HLA and Disease Associations*. Springer, New York.

Uryu, N., Maeda, M., Ota, M., Tsuji, K. and Inoko, H. (1990). A simple and rapid method for HLA-DRB and -DQB typing by digestion of PCR-amplified DNA with allele specific restriction endonucleases. *Tissue Antigens* **35**: 20–31.

Woolf, B. (1955). On estimating the relation between blood group and disease. *Ann. Hum. Genet.* **19**: 251–253.

Yang, S.Y. (1987). A standardised method for the detection of HLA-A and HLA-B alleles by one-dimensional isoelectric focussing (IEF) gel electrophoresis. In *Immunobiology of HLA, Volume I, Histocompatibility Testing 1987* (ed. B. Dupont), Springer-Verlag, New York.

Appendix: statistical notes

Discrete and continuous data and probability distributions

The distribution of heights in the population represents an example of a continuous distribution. When one describes someone as 5 ft 9 in, that represents an approximation suggesting the height lies somewhere between 5 ft 8.5 in and 5 ft 9.5 in. If one wished to do so, it would theoretically be possible to allocate individuals to ever more precisely defined categories. By contrast, this would not be possible if you were tabulating the number of children in families in your study population. It has no meaning to aim for more precision in data collection in the latter case. This is an example of discrete data. They can be quantified but there are no intermediate measurements.

In the discussion of the frequency of HLA alleles, we have used phrases such as 'the variable has a normal distribution'. What does that mean in this context? Let us assume we toss a coin. There is an equal chance of it falling as heads or tails. If we toss a coin twice, we can have three results: two heads, two tails or one of each, but it is twice as likely to have one of each. If we plot this as a graph, we would get Figure 6.A1. Extending this to tossing a coin 15 times, we would get the result illustrated in Figure 6.A2. This is beginning to take a shape now – not unlike the shape of a normal distribution. In fact, this distribution is known as the binomial distribution, but at high numbers it approximates to the normal distribution (Figure 6.A3). If we look at Figure 6.A2, it is clear that the mean is 7.5, which is the mean number of heads you would expect if you tossed a coin 15 times. In practice this means in most series you will get 6, 7, 8 or 9 heads. However, in a few series of 15 tosses you will get 5 or 10 heads, in fewer still 4 or 11, and occasionally 3 or less or 12 or more. Exactly the same can be said of the frequencies of HLA antigens. If it is known that an allele is present in 20% of a defined population, then the allele frequency observed in most samples of individuals from within that population will fall into a reasonably narrow range centred around 20%, but the results of a few studies will be rather

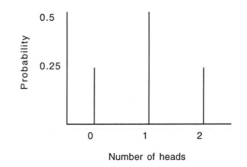

Figure 6.A1 Probability distribution of obtaining a certain number of heads on tossing a coin twice.

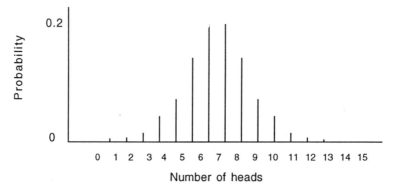

Figure 6.A2 Probability distribution of obtaining a certain number of heads on tossing a coin 15 times.

different. If you perform an analysis of the frequency of that antigen in a sample of the same population, the figure you observe can be said to be taken from a normally distributed population of frequencies.

How the chi-square test works

The chi-square test addresses the question: do the sets of observed data under comparison come from the same or from different populations? It is assumed that each of the variables concerned has a normal distribution (Figure 6.A3). All normal

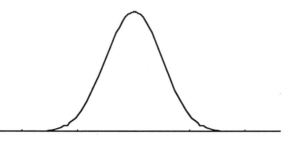

Figure 6.A3 The shape of a normal distribution.

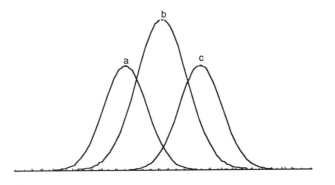

Figure 6.A4   Normal distributions differ from each other in two respects: graphs a and b differ in their means and scale, graphs a and c differ in only their means.

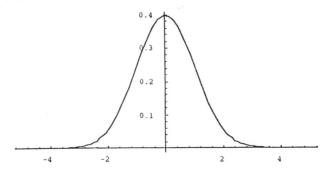

Figure 6.A5   The standard normal distribution.

distributions have the same shape, but they differ from one another in two respects: the value of the mean and the scale (see Figure 6.A4). In order to compare like with like in the same test, all the data have to be 'standardized'. In other words, all data are transformed in such a way that they conform with the particular normal distribution illustrated in Figure 6.A5, the 'standard normal distribution', which has a mean of 0 and a standard deviation of 1.

The statistic used to generate the data in the chi-square test $(O-E)^2/E$, involves O, the observed value, and E, the expected value, which would be the mean of the population if all the data came from the same population. $(O-E)^2/E$ approximates all the data to a standard normal distribution to allow comparison. First, all data are standardized to a mean of zero. If the observed number is the same as the population mean, $O-E$ is equal to zero. If it is not, the expression $O-E$ is a measure of the deviation of the observed value from the mean (Figure 6.A6). This deviation may be positive or negative. Since we are interested in accumulating deviations, each deviation is squared in order to make all the numbers positive. In this way, with each additional measure of deviation, the cumulative total increases. For example, in Figure 6.A6, the sum of a (-1) and b (2) would be 1, but the sum of a^2 (1) and b^2 (4) would be 5.

By dividing it by E, the second standardization is effected. This may be explained by this example. If you found one giraffe was an inch taller than another, you would not be surprised. However, if one caterpillar was an inch longer than another, the

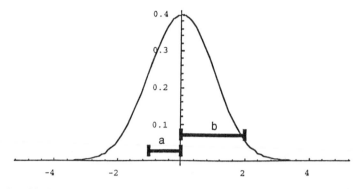

Figure 6.A6 Graphical representation of deviations within standard normal distribution.

difference would be very striking. You could quantify the relative significance of the inch difference by dividing by the average height of a giraffe or the average length of a caterpillar. This would show that the deviation from the norm is much greater for the caterpillar.

The 'chi-square distribution with one degree of freedom' (Figure 6.A7) is a distribution of the standardized squared deviations from the mean of a variable with a standard normal distribution, of which $(O-E)^2/E$ is an approximation. What does that distribution mean? Assume there was one point in the centre of every square millimetre box under the normal distribution curve in Figure 6.A3. If you calculated the variance for each of these points and plotted them on a graph of size against number of points the graph would look like that in Figure 6.A7.

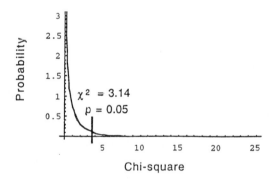

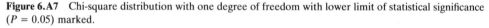

Figure 6.A7 Chi-square distribution with one degree of freedom with lower limit of statistical significance ($P = 0.05$) marked.

In the chi-square test, we can add standardized variances for several independent variables. The sequence of graphs in Figure 6.A8 shows the distributions obtained when we add together variances from a number of independent variables. It is important to know how many independent variables we are dealing with which is what is referred to as the number of degrees of freedom. This is discussed below.

As with other statistical tests, if the observed result is likely to arise by chance in only a small percentage of situations, a more acceptable explanation is that the data being compared do not come from the same population. This is what is meant by there being a statistically significant difference between them. For the chi-square distributions, the figure above which 5% of values of χ^2 occur (i.e. $P<0.05$) increases with the number of degrees of freedom (Figure 6.A7). Some of these data are tabulated in Table 6.5.

Degrees of freedom

As noted above, the number of degrees of freedom is another way of referring to the number of independent variables involved. This is usually one less than the total number of variables. This can be explained as follows. In our 2×2 contingency table, we define an individual as being $DR2^+$ or $DR2^-$. These are not independent conditions. If someone is $DR2^+$, they cannot also be $DR2^-$. Hence there is only one independent variable. Similarly, each individual is either a patient or a control. In a contingency table, the total number of degrees of freedom is the product of the degrees of freedom for the rows and those of the columns [i.e. $(n-1)(m-1)$]. If one were looking at five different independent phenotypic markers in patients and controls, the number of degrees of freedom would be $(5-1)(2-1) = 4 \times 1 = 4$.

It is important to consider the independence of the variable. In a study of a diallelic locus, it may be of interest to examine the associations with the three possible genotypes: AA, Aa and aa. Initial impressions might be that any such study would involve two degrees of freedom. However, given the gene frequency of either A or a, it is possible to calculate the other, and with it the frequency of AA, Aa and aa. Therefore, this constitutes only one degree of freedom.

The Yates' continuity correction

The Yates' continuity correction for small samples helps make the discrete data generated by the test statistic, $\Sigma(O-E)^2/E$, more closely approximate to the chi-squared distribution. With the correction, the statistic calculated is $\Sigma(|O-E| - 1/2)^2/E$ rather than $\Sigma(O-E)^2/E$.[1] This may be explained by assuming a discrete distribution over the range 0–20. There will be 20 lines drawn, the first at 1 and the 20th at 20. But a continuous distribution extending over that range will begin at 0. If one were to draw the axis of symmetry for each of these distributions, it would be at 10 for the continuous distribution but at 10.5 for the discrete distribution. The two are brought more closely into line by subtracting 0.5 of an interval from each of the data. In essence, one is assuming that the data at, say, point 10, actually represents the data in the range $9<x\leqslant10$, and plotting it at 9.5.

Yates' correction is only important at small sample sizes but some statisticians believe it is needlessly conservative.

Fisher's exact test

This test is valuable when expected frequencies in a 2×2 contingency table are too low for a chi-square test to be applicable.

---

[1] Flanking a number or expression with vertical lines indicates 'modulus'. This means the number is represented without a sign. Positive numbers are unchanged and negative numbers are altered to their positive equivalent.

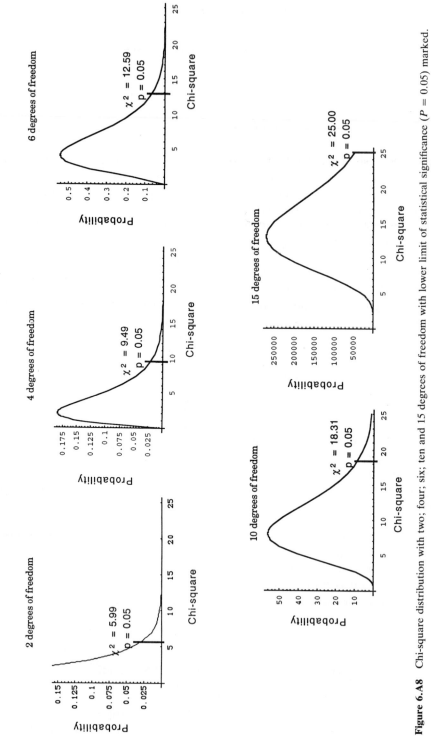

Figure 6.A8 Chi-square distribution with two; four; six; ten and 15 degrees of freedom with lower limit of statistical significance ($P = 0.05$) marked.

To explain the principle of the test we shall use an example of a fictitious study that is clearly too small to be of value in practice.

	DR2⁻ individuals	DR2⁺ individuals	Totals
Disease	1	3	**4**
Controls	2	2	**4**
Totals	**3**	**5**	**8**

The null hypothesis states that there is no association between this disease and DR2.

Fisher's exact test asks this question: given the four totals (shown in bold in the table), what is the likelihood that this combination of figures arose by chance? In fact there are only four possible ways of filling in the gaps in this table, since there are only four possible figures that can be inserted into the DR2⁻ disease box: 0, 1, 2, 3 – all other figures follow from that.

	DR2⁻ individuals	DR2⁺ individuals	Totals
Disease			**4**
Controls			**4**
Totals	**3**	**5**	**8**

The four possibilities are outlined below:

(A)

	DR2⁻	DR2⁺	Totals
Disease	0	4	4
Controls	3	1	4
Totals	3	5	8

(B)

	DR2⁻	DR2⁺	Totals
Disease	1	3	4
Controls	2	2	4
Totals	3	5	8

(C)

	DR2⁻	DR2⁺	Totals
Disease	2	2	4
Controls	1	3	4
Totals	3	5	8

(D)

	DR2⁻	DR2⁺	Totals
Disease	3	1	4
Controls	0	4	4
Totals	3	5	8

Let us label the eight subjects a–h, and call the DR2⁻ subjects a, b and c, and the DR2⁺ individuals d–h. What are the possible combinations in each of these tables? In tables A and D, subjects a, b and c are committed to a single box; the single individual in the DR2⁺/control box is one and only one of the others: thus there are five possible permutations of each of tables A and D. Tables B and C similarly have identical numbers of permutations: the numbers in the two rows have merely been swapped. In table B, the DR2⁻/disease subject could be a, b or c (three possibilities). There are ten possible combinations of d, e, f, g and h to make up the trio in the

DR2[+]/disease box: def, deg, deh, dfg, dfh, dgh, efg, efh, egh and fgh. The total number of permutations for each of tables B and C is thus $3 \times 10 = 30$. Add to this the 5 for each of tables A and D, and the total number of permutations for these tables is 70. From this it is possible to work out the possibility of each table arising:

Table	Probability	
A	5/70 =	0.071
B	30/70 =	0.429
C	30/70 =	0.429
D	5/70 =	0.071

The observed data conformed to table B, which has a probability of occurring by chance of 0.429. Hence the null hypothesis stands and it is not possible to infer an association between DR2 and this disease from these data. In fact, none of the possible tables for these data had a probability of occurring less than 0.05, so no combination of figures with these row and column totals could have given a statistically significant association using Fisher's exact test. However, it is clear that almost any more complex table or one with larger numbers is likely to have one or more combinations that would occur by chance only rarely. This illustrates the potential of this approach. In practice, Fisher's exact test is applied by entering the data into an appropriate computer program.

Relative risk and significance testing

The statistical significance of a relative risk (RR) can be calculated using the chi-square distribution. Using the nomenclature of Table 6.7, we first calculate the variance using the formula:

$$V = 1/a + 1/b + 1/c + 1/d \tag{6.A1}$$

Next, the test statistic is calculated using this expression:

$$(1/V) \times (\log_e RR)^2 \tag{6.A2}$$

The value obtained is then compared with the chi-square distribution for one degree of freedom. As before, to obtain statistical significance ($P < 0.05$) the test statistic must be > 3.84.

For small values of a, b, c or d, Haldane has introduced a modification of the formula to calculate RR (Haldane, 1956).

$$RR = \frac{(2a+1)(2d+1)}{(2b+1)(2c+1)} \tag{6.A3}$$

The variance for significance testing is calculated according to the following formula:

$$V = 1/(a+1) + 1/(b+1) + 1/(c+1) + 1/(d+1) \tag{6.A4}$$

This is discussed further in Tiwari and Terasaki (1985).

Lod scores

An alternative method of assessing linkage between an HLA allele and a disease susceptibility locus (and, indeed, of quantifying the closeness of the linkage) is the method of log odds ratios or 'lod scores'. A detailed explanation of the mathematics involved is provided in Cavalli-Sforza and Bodmer (1971). The following explanation is based on their discussion.

Figure 6.A9 represents the pedigree of a family in which a number of individuals have hereditary elliptocytosis (filled rather than empty symbols). In this figure, each individual's rhesus blood group is presented to allow us to study the possibility of linkage between rhesus phenotype and elliptocytosis. The three rhesus genotypes within the family are designated A, B and C. It can be predicted that, if there is no linkage between elliptocytosis and rhesus phenotype, 50% of the affected progeny would have maternal rhesus genotype A and 50%, C. Conversely, if the two phenotypes are so closely linked that there are no recombination events between them, then all the affected progeny would have the same rhesus phenotype. The probability of the observed pedigree arising in either the case of non-linkage or non-recombination, as well as all intermediate levels of linkage may be calculated. It is therefore possible to obtain the value for linkage (θ) (percentage recombination between the two loci) that gives the maximum probability of obtaining the observed pedigree.

In this example, the value which gives the maximum probability of obtaining the observed pedigree is 0.11, or an 11% recombination frequency. The log odds ratio (or z, the lod score) is a ratio of this probability divided by the probability of obtaining this pedigree if there were no linkage. In our example, with a value of q of 0.11, the formula gives a z value of 1.044 which is the logarithm of the ratio of odds 11:1. In other words, there is an 11 to 1 odds in favour of linkage between rhesus blood groups and elliptocytosis. Does this constitute significance? As with all statistical tests, it is somewhat arbitrary where one draws the line between significance and non-significance. Tiwari and Terasaki (1985) suggest significance levels of 1000 to 1 ($z = +3.000$) and 100 to 1 ($z = -2.00$) for positive and negative linkages, respectively.

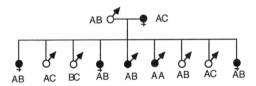

Figure 6.A9 Sample pedigree for method of lod scores. See discussion in text.

CHAPTER 7
HLA and autoimmune disease

Robert Heard
Department of Neurology
Royal Prince Alfred Hospital
Sydney, Australia

Introduction

Autoimmunity

The ability to discriminate accurately between self and non-self is critical to the performance of a competent immune system, which is required to respond in a highly specific manner to foreign antigens yet at the same time remain unresponsive to often highly immunogenic self antigens. This phenomenon of self tolerance, originally given the name *horror autoxicus* by Paul Ehrlich, unfortunately is not immutable and can break down. *Autoimmunity* describes a process in which an individual's immune system becomes sensitized to self antigens, and frequently this results in the development of a pathological state. There are over 40 diseases of man which are known to be caused by autoimmune processes (Tiwari and Terasaki, 1985). These diseases, which can involve any part of the body, include such major causes of morbidity as insulin-dependent diabetes mellitus (IDDM), rheumatoid arthritis (RA), multiple sclerosis (MS), myasthenia gravis (MG), systemic lupus erythematosus (SLE), and autoimmune thyroiditis. Together, autoimmune diseases affect more than 5% of the population. Despite their apparently diverse nature, it is believed that in each of these diseases the propagation of the autoimmune response is the result of similar immunological mechanisms, raising for the first time the tantalizing possibility that all autoimmune disease might become treatable by specific immune intervention in the foreseeable future.

Human autoimmune disease may be classified in several ways. A fundamental distinction appears to exist between the organ-specific autoimmune diseases and the non-organ-specific, or multi-system, autoimmune diseases. The former are characterized by an immune response directed against a single tissue or protein. Many of the

HLA and Disease
ISBN 0–12–440320–4

best examples of this are endocrine diseases such as IDDM, thyroiditis, Addison's disease, and primary gonadal failure, in which there is destruction of a particular secretory cell type. Other diseases, of which MS is an example, are thought likely to be organ-specific despite the fact that a target antigen has not yet been positively identified. Multi-system autoimmune diseases, such as RA, SLE, and the other connective tissue diseases, appear to be rather different and are associated with a variety of autoantibodies against ubiquitous cytoplasmic and nuclear molecules involved in cellular replication.

Autoimmunity can result in cellular damage through several mechanisms. In organ-specific diseases such as IDDM there is attack by both activated T-cells and by autoantibodies, resulting in loss of cells and eventually a corresponding loss of normal physiological function. Autoantibodies directed against a receptor may result in decreased function, as with anti-acetylcholine receptor antibodies in MG (Hohlfeld et al. 1985), or they may stimulate the receptor by mimicking some of the effects of the ligand, as in the case of Graves' disease (Adams, 1958). The multi-system autoimmune diseases are also mediated by both T-cells and by antibodies. In RA for instance, abnormal T-cell activation is detected in synovial fluid of affected joints, and a variety of autoantibodies are also found in high titres (Zvaifler, 1988). In SLE and polyarteritis nodosa (PAN) the deposition of circulating immune complexes in the walls of blood vessels is a potent trigger of more destructive autoimmune reactivity (Theofilopoulos and Dixon, 1981).

The association between autoimmune diseases and HLA

It has become clear that the fundamental property of HLA molecules is their ability to bind peptide fragments and present these to antigen receptors on the surface of T-cells. Class II molecules of the MHC act as co-recognition elements, with foreign antigen, by CD4-positive T-cells. MHC class II molecules also determine the immune response phenotype to a large number of antigens, and stimulate auto- and allo-mixed lymphocyte reactions, as discussed in Chapters 3 and 4. These functions account for the pivotal role played by MHC class II molecules in T-cell-dependent immune responses. This gives us a theoretical basis for equivalent MHC restriction in the case of auto-antigens, raising the possibility that class II alleles might be true susceptibility genes for autoimmune diseases, and providing a major impetus for studies of MHC genes in autoimmunity. Susceptibility to almost all autoimmune diseases is influenced by genes encoded within the MHC. Whilst the earliest studies were able to demonstrate that many human diseases are associated to varying degrees with class I alleles, it has become apparent as a result of improved techniques for analysing the MHC region that in autoimmune diseases class II antigens are more important. The MHC class I-associated diseases, particularly the HLA B27-associated spondylo-arthropathies such as ankylosing spondylitis (AS) and Reiter's syndrome, are much less frequent. This chapter will concentrate therefore on the role played by the genes of the class II region in autoimmune disease, although AS will also be discussed. Present concepts have derived from three areas of study. Firstly, a great many diseases have been found to be associated with HLA alleles, and these associations are especially strong in the case of diseases with a definite or likely autoimmune pathogenesis (Svejgaard et al., 1983; Tiwari and Terasaki, 1985). Conversely, in almost all class II-associated diseases, autoimmune phenomena can be demonstrated. Whilst the majority of these data have linked disease susceptibility with individual alleles, some studies have raised the possibility that risk is further increased by heterozygosity, and there are also instances where it is the combination of alleles on a given extended haplotype which may be important. Secondly, the elucidation of large numbers of human and murine class II gene sequences has led to the identification of nucleotide substitutions which are associated very closely with susceptibility and resistance to disease. Lastly, data from experimental animal models of autoimmune diseases (as discussed below) have confirmed that class II antigens can alone determine susceptibility and resistance to the disease in particular strains.

The rate of progress of determining the association between MHC and disease has been limited by our ability to characterize accurately the HLA system. Tissue typing was first carried out, and still is, using polyclonal antisera. While this method allows considerable polymorphism to be detected at the class I loci, the class II loci such as DQ were not so easily typed. Many other techniques are now in routine use, and much effort has been put into correlating the results obtained by each of them. The expressed class II gene products can now be detected by means of class- and allele-specific monoclonal antibodies, by T-cell alloreactivity (in the mixed lymphocyte reaction and by clonal T-cell responses), and by electrophoretic analysis of immuno-precipitated α and β chains. Polymorphism in the class II region can also be studied at the genetic level, by analysis of restriction fragment length polymorphism (RFLP), by enzymatic amplification of a gene followed by either hybridization with sequence-specific oligonucleotide probes (SSO) or by digestion of the amplified gene with a panel of restriction enzymes, and by direct nucleotide sequence analysis. HLA-typing techniques were discussed in greater detail in Chapter 6. The sequences of the majority of common alleles of DP, DQ and DR are now known (Horn et al., 1988).

The first recorded associations of human disease with an HLA antigen were those of Hodgkin's lymphoma with a cross-reactive group of antigens, HLA-B5, B35, B15 and B18 (Amiel, 1967), and acute lymphoblastic leukaemia with HLA-A2 (Walford et al., 1970). At the same time, the demonstration by McDevitt and Benacerraf (1969) that murine immune responses were controlled by MHC-linked genes led to early attempts to establish the relationship between the HLA system and human autoimmune disease. Soon afterwards the extremely strong association between ankylosing spondylitis and HLA-B27 was discovered (Brewerton et al., 1973; Schlosstein et al., 1973). This provided an early impetus for further research into the disease associa-tions of both class I and class II antigens, and there is now an enormous literature describing these studies. The known HLA and disease associations have been comprehensively reviewed by Tiwari and Terasaki (1985). Some of the more important associations of autoimmune disease with class I and class II antigens are shown in Table 7.1. It can be seen that almost without exception, these diseases are most strongly associated with the class II antigen HLA DR. Associations between class II genotype and susceptibility to more than 40 different autoimmune diseases have been reported. In each of these diseases there is strong circumstantial evidence that the immune system reacts against particular self antigens. In animal models of autoimmunity, such as experimental allergic encephalomyelitis (EAE) and experimental allergic myasthenia gravis (EAMG), the autoantigen is known and can be fully characterized. However, this is true of only a few of the human autoimmune diseases and in most cases the autoantigen towards which the destructive immune response is

Table 7.1 The predominant HLA-DR associations of human diseases with definite or probable autoimmune pathogenesis

Disease	Associated antigen	Relative risk
Rheumatoid arthritis	DR4	2–6
	DR1	2–4
Juvenile rheumatoid arthritis	DR5	3
	DRw8	2
Progressive systemic sclerosis	DR5	2
Systemic lupus erythematosus	DR3	2–5
	DR2	2
Insulin-dependent diabetes	DR3	3–6
	DR4	2–7
Graves' disease	DR3	4
	DR5[a]	5–7
Hashimoto's disease	DR3	3
	DR5	2
Vitiligo	DR4	2
Pemphigus vulgaris	DR4	15
	DRw6[b]	5
Psoriasis vulgaris	DR7	3–8
Dermatitis herpetiformis	DR3	17
Coeliac disease	DR3[c,d]	12
	DR7	8
Multiple sclerosis	DR2	2–4
	DR4[e]	12
	DRw6[f]	5
Myasthenia gravis	DR3	2–3
Stiff-man syndrome	n.d.	
Narcolepsy	DR2[g]	130–360
Goodpasture's syndrome	DR2	14

[a] In Japanese.
[b] In non-Ashkenazi Jews.
[c] Relative risk is significantly higher in DR3/7 heterozygotes.
[d] CD may be more strongly associated with DP and DQ than DR (see text).
[e] In Italians and Jordanian arabs.
[f] In Japanese.
[g] See Chapter 9.
n.d. = not yet determined.

directed remains unknown. Some of the better known autoantigens are listed in Table 7.2. In a few cases, there is little or no evidence of a primary immunological process, and yet the strength of the association argues strongly in favour of the HLA antigen itself being the risk factor for disease occurrence, and of it being involved intimately in the pathogenetic process. The most notable example of this is narcolepsy, which is associated with DR2 in virtually 100% of patients (Juji et al., 1984) (see Chapter 9). This has led to speculation that class II antigens may possess important non-immune as well as immune functions (for instance, they may serve as differentiation antigens during embryogenesis), but there is little evidence yet to support this idea.

Class II genes: linked markers or susceptibility genes?

Two forms of relationship between the HLA system and diseases are described. The first is *association*, which is observed as a difference in the frequency of a particular

Table 7.2   Antigens associated with immune responses in human autoimmune diseases[a]

Disease	Associated antigen
Coeliac disease	α-Gliadin
Dermatitis herpetiformis	Unknown
Goodpasture's syndrome	Basement membrane collagen
Graves' disease	TSH receptor
Hashimoto's disease	Thyroglobulin
Insulin-dependent diabetes	Glutamic acid decarboxylase
	Insulin receptor
Multiple sclerosis	Unknown
Myasthenia gravis	Acetyl choline receptor
Narcolepsy	(Mechanism unknown)
Pemphigus vulgaris	'PeV antigen complex'
Progressive systemic sclerosis	DNA topoisomerase
	RNA polymerase
Psoriasis vulgaris	Unknown
Rheumatoid arthritis	Immunoglobulin Fc
Rheumatoid arthritis-juvenile	Immunoglobulin Fc
Stiff-man syndrome	Glutamic acid decarboxylase[b]
Systemic lupus erythematosus	ds-DNA
Vitiligo	Unknown

[a] Autoantibodies are described in most autoimmune diseases. However, in many cases T-cell autoreactivity may be the primary and dominant abnormality (see text).
[b] anti-GAD antibodies in stiff-man syndrome are of higher affinity than those seen in IDDM

allele between affected subjects and healthy controls in population studies. The second is *linkage*, which is detected as a distortion of the expected random pattern of segregation of haplotypes between the members of a family in which there are a number of affected subjects. Frustratingly, in the case of the HLA system and autoimmune diseases, both association and linkage have been observed, but neither is sufficiently strong to account entirely for disease susceptibility. Whereas the absence of disease in healthy subjects possessing a disease-associated haplotype can be accounted for by the lack of a necessary environmental factor, the presence of disease in individuals without the appropriate haplotype is more puzzling. For example, 32% of Caucasian patients with rheumatoid arthritis (RA) do not have DR4, 49% of patients with multiple sclerosis (MS) do not have DR2, and 52% of those with psoriasis vulgaris (PV) do not have DR7 (Tiwari and Terasaki, 1985). The weakness of these associations is probably accounted for in part, but not entirely, by disease heterogeneity. Examples of this include RA, a clinically similar but genetically distinct form of which occurs in children and adolescents; MS which exists in two clinically distinct extremes, primarily chronic progressive and relapsing/remitting (Matthews, 1985); and diabetes mellitus, of which at least three distinct types exist (IDDM, NIDDM and MODY). Another possible explanation for these weak associations is that the class II gene product identified by alloreactive antisera traditionally used in tissue-typing does not exactly represent the disease susceptibility gene itself, but is merely linked to it. In the case of MS, for example, a putative susceptibility gene might be an allele of another locus in tight linkage disequilibrium with DR2 (DQw6 for instance). A further proposal is that susceptibility might be mediated through a class II epitope(s) which results from the co-expression of two or more genes that are commonly associated with the disease-associated haplotype, but which are also found on other haplotypes. Finally, another alternative explanation might be that susceptibility is associated with a casette of amino-acid sequence which is shared by a number of serologically distinct alleles.

This question of whether susceptibility is governed directly by class II genes or by different closely linked genes has been a major issue in understanding autoimmunity. The hope and expectation that improved methods of accurately identifying class II alleles would reveal much closer associations with diseases were not realized, however, until quite recently. Polymorphism within the class II region can be defined by a number of techniques, as described earlier. RFLP analysis in particular enabled a large number of previously unknown class II subspecificities to be identified, and the results of allogenotyping by this method correlate well with the other techniques, as the Tenth International Histocompatibility Workshop data (DuPont, 1989), and more recently sequence analysis of alleles, have clearly shown. The highest hopes were held for allogenotyping by means of RFLP analysis, a technique which lends itself readily to population studies. However, although particular class II restriction fragments *are* associated with diseases, the strengths of these associations have rarely increased substantially above those observed using established serological methods.

Thus RFLP studies were unable to answer the fundamental question, whether the class II genes are themselves susceptibility genes or merely linked genes. The only approach which might be capable of revealing allelic polymorphism not detected by other methods was nucleotide sequence analysis. This approach was made feasible by the application of the polymerase chain reaction (PCR), making it possible to determine the sequences of DR, DQ and DP alleles in large numbers of patients and healthy individuals (Horn et al., 1988; Bugawan et al., 1988). Several groups have now contributed sequence data in a number of different diseases. One of the major conclusions has been that individual specific class II alleles are not associated exclusively with autoimmune diseases but are also present in healthy subjects also. This is consistent with the suggestion that most, if not all, autoimmune diseases are polygenic, and that HLA antigens constitute one of a number of susceptibility factors. In addition, it is possible that the true susceptibility genes remain to be identified. The strengths of many of the HLA-disease associations suggest that a susceptibility gene is either another HLA gene, or a non-HLA gene lying within the MHC and in strong linkage disequilibrium with the HLA marker. The recent discovery of new families of genes centromeric to DQ is fuelling speculation that disease susceptibility genes other than HLA exist within the MHC region (see Chapter 9).

However, for certain diseases, it has also been possible to identify short cassettes of sequence, often represented within more than one class II allele, which are associated with disease susceptibility or resistance. An important breakthrough made in this way was the observation that the amino acid residue at position 57 of the DQβ chain is correlated closely with the risk of developing IDDM (Todd et al., 1987). This finding provides strong evidence that class II genes themselves may be concerned directly in determining susceptibility to at least some autoimmune diseases. Disease-associated allelic micropolymorphism has been reported in other diseases, most successfully in the cases of RA and PV.

Non-MHC genes in autoimmunity

Data from many sources indicate that susceptibility to autoimmune diseases is multifactorial and polygenic. It is therefore insufficient to consider the role of the

HLA genes in isolation. Recent studies have demonstrated that the T-cell antigen receptor is also intimately involved in disease susceptibility. Associations with immunoglobulin allotypes have been reported for several diseases, including auto-immune thyroiditis and MS (Pandey et al., 1981), but generally they are weaker than the associations observed with the HLA system. Many other genetic systems have been incriminated at various times, for example erythrocyte surface antigens, α-1-antitrypsin inhibitor and alkaline phosphatase. The well-known observations that many class II-associated autoimmune diseases are more common in females, and that the HLA B27-associated spondyloarthropathies more common in males, remain unexplained but suggest that hormonal factors influence the pathogenesis of some diseases. There is also evidence linking susceptibility to diabetes in the mouse, and possibly also in man, to the gene encoding the T-cell antigen Thy-1. The recent discovery of ATP-binding cassette transporter genes and some of the proteasome-related genes in the class II region raises alternative explanations for HLA-linked disease susceptibility that can be accounted for by non-HLA genes (see Chapter 9).

The role of environmental factors in autoimmunity

It is accepted now that environmental influences can play an important part in the development of autoimmune disease. This conclusion has been reached from meticulous epidemiological surveys, from reports of disease appearing following a viral infection and being associated with a rise in viral antibody titres, and from the association of some autoimmune diseases with certain drugs or toxins. As an example of the first of these, the relationship between prevalence of MS and latitude in Australia was studied (Hammond et al., 1988). Although it is well established that MS is most common between latitudes 45° and 65°, and less common at equatorial and Mediterranean latitudes, this observation could be accounted for to a large degree by the global distribution of populations of northern European ancestry. However, a rigorous study of European immigrants to Perth (32°S) and Hobart (43°S) clearly demonstrated that the north–south gradient in Australia is not genetically determined, and that environmental factors have modified disease expression. Other examples are numerous. IDDM is occasionally observed to develop following infection with a Coxsackie virus (Yoon et al., 1979). Lymphocytes from HLA B27-positive patients with ankylosing spondylitis are lysed by antibodies to some strains of *Klebsiella* (Grennan and Sanders, 1988). SLE can be precipitated by procainamide and hydrallazine. There is epidemiological evidence linking MS with both measles and canine distemper viruses (Kurtzke, 1980).

However, despite numerous studies implicating specific microorganisms in the aetiology of many autoimmune diseases, attempts to confirm that they have a causative role have been largely unsuccessful. There are a number of possible reasons for this. Firstly, infection with a virus may have been a historical event preceding the onset of autoimmunity by many months or years. The virus may have been entirely eliminated in that time, or it may have become latent in the host, present at extremely low levels in specific tissues. Alternatively, it may be necessary for a genetically susceptible individual to have been infected with two or more different viruses before an autoimmune process is triggered. In many instances it is the very weakness of both the genetic and the environmental associations of autoimmune

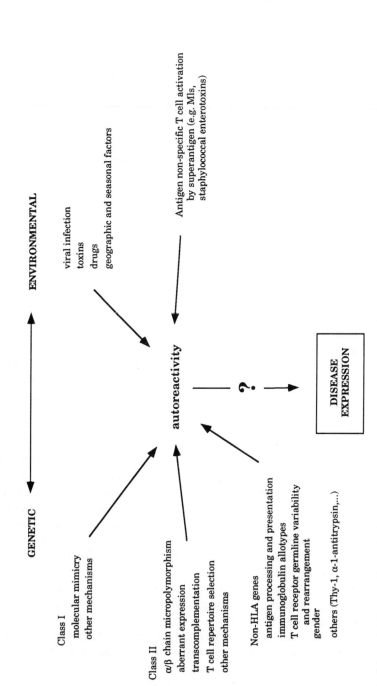

Figure 7.1 Schematic diagram illustrating some of the possible genetic and environmental factors responsible for the development of autoreactivity and autoimmune disease.

diseases which underlines the importance of the interrelationships between the two, as portrayed somewhat schematically in Figure 7.1.

HLA and autoimmune diseases

In this section the relationship of six important human diseases with the HLA system will be discussed. IDDM and RA are major causes of morbidity, and MS is the commonest cause of neurological disability in young people. There is good evidence that each of these diseases involves autoimmune mechanisms, particularly in the case of IDDM. Pemphigus vulgaris (PeV) and coeliac disease (CD) are also discussed, as they shed further light on the role that MHC class II antigens may play in autoimmunity. The final disease discussed here will be ankylosing spondylitis (AS), which has a spectacular association with the class I antigen B27, and which serves to illustrate that there is unlikely to be a single pathogenetic mechanism underlying the whole spectrum of autoimmunity.

Insulin-dependent diabetes mellitus

IDDM is an autoimmune disease in which there is destruction of the β cells of the islets of Langerhans in the pancreas, resulting in the impaired production of insulin. Histologically there is infiltration of the islets with large numbers of inflammatory cells including T and B lymphocytes, and MHC class II expression occurs on the β cells (Bottazzo et al., 1985). Autoantibodies to both islet cells and insulin are present, and often can be detected long before the appearance of diabetes (Srikanta et al., 1983). It has been proposed that aberrant expression of MHC class II molecules on islet cells could be an initiating event, and until recently this hypothesis has been favoured widely (Campbell and Harrison, 1990). The hypothesis that aberrant MHC class II expression provides a trigger for autoimmunity was discussed in Chapter 4. This hypothesis has had a further set-back following the recent discovery that MHC class II molecules in non-obese diabetic (NOD) mice are expressed only on cells of lymphoid origin, and that neither class II nor ICAM-1 are expressed on the surface of β-cells (McInerney et al., 1991; O'Reilly et al., 1991). Both these studies demonstrated increased expression of class I on the β-cells, however, suggesting that this may play a role in immunopathogenesis, and clearly this is an important area for future studies.

   Many lines of evidence suggest that IDDM is a multi-factorial disease, triggered by environmental factors in genetically susceptible individuals. The environmental trigger is unknown, although there is some evidence that infection with any of a number of viruses, including rubella, Coxsackie, mumps and cytomegalovirus, may precede the appearance of the disease (Vague, 1984). There is equally strong evidence that IDDM is in part genetically determined, although the mode of inheritance has not been established. IDDM has a concordance rate in monozygotic twins of 30–50%, substantially higher than for most other autoimmune diseases, and a significantly increased risk among other first degree relatives. In the NOD mouse there appear to be at least three diabetogenic loci, one in the MHC (possibly H-2Ab), a T-cell antigen

(Thy-1) encoded on chromosome 9, and one at present unidentified. There have been two attempts to map IDDM susceptibility to the human Thy-1 gene, which is located on chromosome 11, with inconclusive results. In one RFLP study there was a significant association between IDDM and the CD3e allele lying on chromosome 11q23 but in females only (Wong et al., 1991). In a study of 81 multiplex IDDM families the presence of a susceptibility gene was excluded throughout more than 90% of the homologous region on 11q (Hyer et al., 1991). The presence of non-HLA susceptibility genes in the MHC region is a possibility which, as mentioned elsewhere, has received much impetus from the discovery of the ABC-transporter genes and some proteosome-related genes (see Chapter 9). There have already been two long-range mapping studies of the HLA region in IDDM (Christiansen et al., 1990; Niven et al., 1990). The first of these studies found evidence for deletions in diabetogenic DR3 ancestral haplotypes which were not present in non-diabetogenic haplotypes, although in the Niven study there were no differences between diabetic and non-diabetic individuals.

Population studies

Clear evidence of genetically determined susceptibility to IDDM has come from studies of HLA markers in both populations and families. The first described associations were with HLA B8, B18 and B15, but a more significant association was later observed with the class II specificities DR3 and DR4 (Tiwari and Terasaki, 1985). Ninety-five per cent of Caucasoid patients possess either HLA DR3 or DR4, compared to 45–54% of healthy individuals. Susceptibility is associated particularly with the DR4/Dw4/DQw8 haplotype and with the DR3/Dw3/Dw24/DQw2 haplotype. Two other Caucasian haplotypes are also positively associated with IDDM, DR1/DQw5 and DR2/DQw5/DwAZH. Certain haplotypes are observed at reduced frequency in IDDM, and are therefore thought to be protective. The most important of these is DR2/Dw2/DQw6, but DR4/DQw7 and DR5/DQw7 are also associated with negative risk (Ilonen et al., 1978; Thomsen et al., 1979). Other haplotypes are neutral and confer no risk. DR3 and DR4 are associated with IDDM in all populations studied, whereas in Japanese and Chinese patients, but not in Caucasoids, DRw9 appears to be increased (Aparicio et al., 1988).

   The individual risks of DR3 and DR4 are not simply additive, and the risk of developing IDDM is further increased in DR3/4 heterozygotes (Nerup 1978; Wolf et al., 1983). Deschamps, in a large study of IDDM patients and controls (Deschamps et al., 1988), has investigated the distortions in the expected gene frequencies on extended haplotypes, for both *cis* (same haplotype) and *trans* (opposite haplotype) loci. It was found that in the *trans* situation there was a large excess of DR3/4 heterozygotes (RR = 51, $P < 10^{-6}$), and a deficit of DR$x/x$ (RR = 0.12, $P < 10^{-6}$).[1] DR3 and DR4 homozygosity did not differ between patients and controls. Furthermore, a significantly increased frequency of DR1 and C4B*0 in non-DR3, non-DR4 diabetic haplotypes was seen. These findings indicate that transcomplementation may contribute to the development of some autoimmune responses, a possibility which will be discussed below.

---

[1] x in DR x/x indicates a DR specificity other than DR3 or DR4.

Family studies

There have been many reported studies of HLA allele frequencies in IDDM families. These studies have established unequivocally the association with DR3 and DR4, and also the higher relative risk for DR3/DR4 heterozygotes. Analyses by several authors of HLA haplotypes in affected sib-pairs have demonstrated a highly significant distortion of the predicted patterns of segregation (Ryder et al., 1979). This indicates that IDDM and alleles of the HLA system segregate jointly, and support the hypothesis that there is at least one major IDDM susceptibility gene in the MHC. However, attempts to deduce the mode of inheritance from family studies have yielded conflicting results. Data have variously been interpreted as suggesting: (1) a single gene effect with recessive (Rubinstein et al., 1976), dominant (Spielman et al., 1979) or intermediate (Morton et al., 1983) patterns of inheritance; (2) a two-gene effect, involving either two HLA-linked genes (Deschamps et al., 1980) or a single HLA gene and another non-HLA gene (Thomson, 1980); (3) a three-gene effect; or (4) an epistatic model in which a non-HLA gene interacts with HLA genes (Suarez et al., 1979).

RFLP studies

There have been several studies of class II RFLP in IDDM in attempts to define subtypes of DR3 and DR4 more closely associated with the disease than their corresponding serospecificities. These RFLP studies have been helpful in mapping DR4-associated susceptibility to the DQB1 gene, but less helpful in the case of DR3. Although many of these studies have used different terminologies, most of them have shown a significantly increased frequency of DQB1 RFLP patterns associated with the DQw3.2 (DQw8) allele (Cohen-Haguenauer et al., 1985; Festenstein et al., 1986; Nepom et al., 1986; Sachs et al., 1987; Gogolin et al., 1989; Robinson et al., 1989a). A DQB1 association has also been found in non-Caucasian subjects, notably Indians (Serjeantson et al., 1987) and Japanese (Aparicio et al., 1988), although it now appears that the primary disease association in Japanese is with the DQA1 locus rather than the DQB1 locus (see below). There is a single report of a DR3-linked DQA1 RFLP being associated with IDDM in Caucasoids (Carrier et al., 1989).

Similarly the presence of negatively associated haplotypes has been confirmed by RFLP analyses, and this protection in many cases has also been mapped to the DQB1 gene. The relationship between IDDM risk and alleles of DQB1 are shown in Table 7.3.

RFLP studies have further strengthened the case for susceptibility to IDDM being enhanced by heterozygosity. In several studies the co-presence of allelic patterns of DQB1 restriction fragments are associated with disease more strongly than is DR3/4 heterozygosity detected serologically (Michelson and Lernmark, 1987). A popular explanation for this finding is transcomplementation, that is a synergism between two specific haplotypes so as to provide a level of susceptibility greater than the additive risks of each of the haplotypes alone. Nepom et al. (1987) have analysed HLA-DQ heterodimers in IDDM patients by two-dimensional gel electrophoresis, observing the presence of both *cis*- and *trans*-associated molecules, and in particular a *trans*-associated dimer consisting of DQα(DR3) and DQβ(DR4). Recently, a significant excess of DR4/DRw8 heterozygotes has been reported among IDDM patients also

(Ronningen et al., 1989a). This excess was at first detected by serological typing, and when the DQB1 alleles were subsequently determined by RFLP analysis and allele-specific oligonucleotide hybridization analysis, it was found that eight of nine DR4/DRw8 patients were DR4,DQw8/DRw8,DQw4 heterozygotes.

Molecular genetics

The most direct evidence yet for autoimmune disease susceptibility mapping to the HLA D-region has come from sequencing DQ genes in IDDM. Todd et al. (1987, 1988a) cloned and sequenced the gene segments encoding the first domains of DRβ, DQα and DQβ chains from a number of common haplotypes, associated variously with positive, neutral, or negative risk. Several representative haplotypes are shown in Table 7.3. The DR4/DQw8 haplotype confers the highest risk, irrespective of racial group, followed closely by the DR3/DQw2 haplotype. Two other haplotypes are also positively associated with IDDM, DR1/DQw5 and DR2/DQw5/DwAZH. Haplotypes which are associated with negative risk are DR4/DQw7, DR5/DQw7 and particularly

Table 7.3   The relationship between DRB1, DQB1 and DQA1 alleles, the amino acid at position 57 of the DQβ (I-Aβ) chain and the observed risk of IDDM.

	DRB1	DQB1	DQβ57	DQA1	Susc.
Caucasian	DR1	DQw5	Val	A1	+
	DR2	DQw5	Ser	A1	+
	DR2	DQw6	Asp	A1	−
	DR3	DQw2	Ala	A4	+
	DR4	DQw7	Asp	A3	−
	DR4	DQw8	Ala	A3	+
	DR5	DQw7	Asp	A4	0
	DR6(w13)	DQw6	Val	A1	+
	DR6(w13)	DQw6	Asp	A1	−
	DR7	DQw2	Ala	A2	0
	DRw8	DQw4	Asp	A4	0
	DR9	DQw9	Asp	A3	0
Negro	DR2	DQw6	Asp	A1	−
	DR3	DQw2	Ala	A4	+
	DR4	DQw8	Ala	A3	+
	DR6(w13)	DQw6	Asp	A1	−
	DR7	DQw2	Ala	A3	+
	DR7	DQw2	Ala	A2	0
		DQw4			0
		DQW9			0
Japanese	DR1	DQw5	Val	A1	+
	DR4	DQw8	Asp	A3	−
	DR4	DQw7	Asp		−
		DQw4			+
		DQw9			+
	DR6	DQw6	Ala	A1	+
Mouse	NOD	Ab^{NOD}	Ser		+
	ILI	Ab^{NOD}	Ser		−
	CTS	Ab^{NOD}	Ser		−
	B10	Ab	Asp		−
Rat	BB	Susc.	Ser		+
	BB	Res.	Ser		−

DR2/DQw6. Other haplotypes are neutral and confer no risk. When the translated DQB1 sequences from 17 haplotypes were examined it was found that in almost every case, disease risk was associated with the presence of a non-charged amino acid at position 57, whereas haplotypes associated with neutral or negative risk encoded negatively charged aspartate at that position (Asp-57). Several other studies have now confirmed these findings (Horn et al., 1988; Morel et al., 1988; Ronningen et al., 1989b). Remarkably this association extended to the NOD mouse, which possesses an unique Aβ chain (see below) in having a serine at position 57, other non-diabetic strains having Asp-57. Since the NOD mouse does not express H-2E molecules, these data suggest that in this model, it is the Aβ chain which is associated with the autoimmune process (Todd et al., 1988b). In a follow up study of Caucasian multiple case IDDM families, it was found that DQB alleles encoding DQβ Asp-57 were significantly increased in frequency among non-diabetic haplotypes, and that non-Asp-57 DQB alleles were significantly increased among diabetic haplotypes (Morel et al., 1988). It was also found that 96% of the diabetic probands were homozygous non-Asp/non-Asp compared to 19.5% of healthy unrelated controls, giving a relative risk (RR) of 107. In most studies, the results suggest that the protection afforded by DQβ Asp-57 appears to be dominant.

The strength of the DQβ-IDDM relationship in humans raises the possibility that IDDM autoreactive T-cells are recognizing an islet-cell antigen in association with a limited number of DQ molecules (particularly DQw8 and DQw2). From the predicted structure of a class II molecule discussed in Chapter 2 (Brown et al., 1988) it appears that amino acid 57 is directed inwards to the antigen-binding cleft. It is a further possibility that Asp-57 may form a salt bridge with a conserved Arg residue at position 79 of the DQα chain, occluding one end of the cleft. It therefore seems reasonable to predict that an Ala–Asp substitution at position 57 might alter the structure of the DQαβ dimer in such a way as to affect antigen binding and/or T-cell recognition. Evidence that DQβ position 57 is likely to be of functional importance has been provided by Lundin et al. (1988) who have reported the successful generation of CD4-positive T-cell clones which respond only to DQ molecules containing Ala-57. It has also been possible to produce monoclonal antibodies which can detect single amino-acid substitutions at position 57 of the DQβ chain (Atar et al., 1989). In the NOD mouse, immune responsiveness to a variety of antigens appears to be influenced by H-2Aβ, and furthermore the onset of diabetes in this strain can be prevented by treating young pre-diabetic mice with an anti-H-2Aβ chain-specific monoclonal antibody (Singh et al., 1990). Susceptibility to experimental diabetes, induced by the administration of low-dose streptozotocin, is also under H-2A control. Mouse strains possessing H-2A^b or H-2A^k are highly susceptible, whereas those with H-2A^d or H-2A^s are relatively resistant (Tanaka et al., 1990). This observation not only demonstrates that susceptibility to diabetes is under genetic control, but once again highlights the omnipresence of genetic and environmental interplay in initiating autoimmune processes.

Despite this compelling evidence, a number of observations challenge this simple DQβ position-57 model of susceptibility to IDDM. Firstly, certain haplotypes, particularly DR7/DQw2 in Caucasoids, confer neutral or negative risk despite having a neutral residue (Ala) at position 57. However, one explanation for this is that the neutral risk of the Asp-57-negative DR7 haplotype is a function of the DQα chain which, in contrast to the DQβ chain, differs between DR3/DQw2 and DR7/DQw2 haplotypes. By studying the association with IDDM of rare haplotypes in black subjects, Todd et al. (1989) have demonstrated that both DQα and DQβ chains (encoded by DQA1 and DQB1 genes) influence susceptibility. Secondly, the model cannot explain the increased risk of DR3/4 individuals relative to those who are DR3/3 and DR4/4, as these are all Asp-57 negative homozygotes. Thirdly, in a comprehensive analysis of DR4 subtypes and DR4-associated DQB1 alleles, Sheehy et al. (1989) found that IDDM was associated equally with DRB1 as with DQB1 alleles, and they proposed that susceptibility is determined by an interaction between certain alleles of each of these two loci. Fourthly, it has been found recently that I-Ab^{NOD} is not, as was previously thought, unique, but is present in identical form in two closely related but non-diabetogenic strains, ILI and CTS (Koide and Yoshida, 1990). Lastly, as Table 7.3 shows, although there are two genetically distinct strains of the Bio Breeding (BB) rat, IDDM-sensitive and IDDM-resistant, both strains have identical first domain class II β-chain sequences with Ser at position 57. In summary therefore, although there is a great deal of evidence in support of a DQβ position 57 model of IDDM susceptibilty and resistance, it now appears likely that the mechanisms involved will be much more complex than was first thought.

Interesting results have come from studies of Japanese patients (Lundin et al., 1989; Yamagata et al., 1989). In this population, the major predisposing haplotypes are DR4 and DR9. The DQw8 allele of the DQB1 gene, which is associated with IDDM susceptibility in Caucasoids, is not increased in frequency in the Japanese patients. DNA sequence analysis has revealed that the Japanese DR4 and DR9 haplotypes have Asp-57-encoding DQB1 alleles, in contrast to the Caucasian haplotypes, and DQβ Asp-57 was seen at equally high frequencies in both patients and controls. Susceptibility to IDDM in Japanese also appears to differ from that occurring in Caucasians in being more strongly associated with DQA1 rather than DQB1. Todd et al. (1990) have found the DQA1 A3 allele in 96% of patients as opposed to only 53% of controls (RR = 19.7). In summary, genetic susceptibility maps strongly to the MHC region, and in particular to the DQB1 (H-2Ab) locus. However, a simple relationship between susceptibility and allelic micropolymorphism does not, as was hoped until recently, exist and it seems likely that MHC-encoded susceptibility is a function of specific combinations of sequences on one or more locus products, and on one or more haplotype. In order to understand this fully, both structural analyses and functional studies of the class II gene products will be necessary. Meanwhile a desirable goal would be the identification of high-risk family members by means of class II genotyping. When strategies for disease prevention become available it will be possible to target such high-risk individuals for immune intervention.

Rheumatoid arthritis

Rheumatoid arthritis is an inflammatory disease characterized by a chronic synovitis and erosive destruction of the articular surfaces of synovial joints. RA is a clinically heterogeneous disorder, and other tissues are also affected to varying degrees. There is no single diagnostic marker for RA, but a majority of patients have in their blood high titres of rheumatoid factors, autoantibodies that bind the Fc region of autologous IgG. Juvenile chronic arthritis (JCA) is a heterogeneous group of conditions which includes pauciarticular juvenile rheumatoid arthritis (JRA). This is clinically similar to RA but may be genetically quite distinct. Like other autoimmune diseases, RA has a complex, multi-factorial mode of inheritance and it is likely that susceptibility is polygenic (Grennan and Sanders, 1988).

Serological and family studies

The strongest association of RA is with DR4, and this has been seen in almost all populations studied, including Caucasians, American blacks, African blacks, Mexicans, and Japanese (reviewed in Tiwari and Terasaki, 1985). Typically, DR4 is seen in 60–80% of RA patients and in 20% of controls. DR4 can be subdivided by cellular and molecular typing into six subtypes, Dw4, Dw10, Dw13, Dw14, Dw15 and DwKT2, risk being associated particularly with Dw4 and Dw14 subtypes (Nepom et al., 1989; Ollier et al., 1989). Weaker but still significant associations have also been observed with DR1 and DRw10 (Goronzy et al., 1986; Duquesnoy et al., 1984). While seropositive cases of JRA are also associated with DR4, several studies have now shown a strong association also with DR5 and DRw8 (Glass et al., 1980; Fink and Stastny, 1980), and a recent study has highlighted an association with an allele of HLA-DP (DPB2.1) which is independent of previously defined HLA-DR region markers (Begovich et al., 1989). These serological studies have not conclusively shown any association with either the presence or titre of rheumatoid factor, or with the severity of the disease. However, several authors have observed a high frequency of DR3 in RA patients who develop toxic reactions to treatment with penicillamine or gold (Panayi et al., 1978; Gran et al., 1983). Family studies have demonstrated that, as with other HLA-associated autoimmune diseases, there is highly significant haplotype sharing by affected members, suggesting a dominant RA-susceptibility gene linked to HLA (Khan et al., 1979; Nunez et al., 1980). Family studies have also shown a higher concordance rate between monozygotic twins than between HLA-identical siblings (Payami et al., 1986).

The clinical presentation of RA shows considerable diversity, and there is evidence that this diversity is reflected in immunogenetic heterogeneity. Among DR4-positive patients with articular disease only, no additional association is seen with any of DQB1, Dw subtype or C4. This is in contrast with DR4 patients with vasculitis in whom Dw14, DQw7, and C4A null associations are seen, and those with Felty's syndrome in whom DQw7 and C4A null phenotypes are associated (Clarkson et al., 1990; Hillarby et al., 1991). Juvenile rheumatoid arthritis, a clinically similar disease occurring in a younger age group, is associated with DRw8, and in particular with the DRB1 allele *0801 (Melin-Aldana et al., 1990).

Molecular studies

As with IDDM, the recent availability of nucleotide sequences for the majority of the class II alleles has allowed attempts at mapping, at a molecular level, HLA-associated susceptibility in RA. In contrast to IDDM, however, it has been found that the major susceptibility locus for RA is DRB1 rather than DQB1, although as we have seen it is possible that certain DQB alleles may modify the effect of DR4B1 alleles (Lanchbury et al., 1989). By analogy with the correlation of IDDM risk to DQB1 sequences, inspection of the alleles associated with RA shows striking conservation of their amino-acid sequences between positions 65 and 75 in the third hypervariable region (HVR) (Gregersen et al., 1987; Todd et al., 1988a; Nepom et al., 1989). It can be shown that DR4/Dw4 differs from DR4/Dw14, DR4/Dw15 and DR1 in the third HVR by only a single substitution at position 71. As a result of these findings it has been proposed that HLA-associated susceptibility is conferred by the presence of a specific cassette of sequence which may be shared by a number of alleles. In the present example, this hypothesis predicts firstly that DR4 subtypes that differ by non-conservative substitutions in this cassette should not confer susceptibility, and secondly that any less common alleles which contain this cassette might also confer susceptibility. These predictions have been tested and have proved to be correct (Wordsworth et al., 1989). In addition the DR4 Dw subtypes described above, susceptibility is also associated with DR1, which is identical to Dw14 and Dw15, and with DRw10, which differs by only a single additional substitution at position 70. In contrast, the Dw10 and Dw13 subtypes of DR4 have further substitutions at positions 67 (Leu-Ile:Dw10), a more radical charge change at 71 (Arg-Glu:Dw10) and 74 (Ala-Glu:Dw13), respectively. The substitutions at positions 70, 71 and 74 cause a net change in the charge profile of the region, and might be expected to result in significant conformational alteration (Watanabe et al., 1989). It has been reported recently that there is also a significant increase in DRw6 in DR4-negative RA patients (Lang et al., 1990).

It appears likely that the third HVR of the DRβ1 chain is a recognition site for T-cells (Goronzy et al., 1986; Gregersen et al., 1986), and this serves to underline the importance of these data. Recently it has been reported that the DRβ1 amino-acid sequence 70–74 (QKRAA) is also present in Epstein–Barr virus (EBV) gp110; infection with EBV commonly occurs and this could conceivably lead to T-cell recognition of the DRβ1 chain. Moreover a similar degree of sequence homology has been found between DRβ1 and DQw1.2β chains and cytomegalovirus IE2 protein. However, the possibility that an autoimmune response might be initiated in this way remains conjectural at the present time.

Pemphigus vulgaris

Pemphigus vulgaris (PV) is an autoimmune disease of skin and mucosa which is characterized clinically by the formation of blisters. Histologically there is separation of epidermal cells in the basal layer of the epidermis, and the presence of an antibody bound to the intercellular matrix can always be demonstrated. As with myasthenia gravis, the disorder is sometimes seen in association with thymoma. PV occurs in all races but is more common in Jews (Ahmed, 1980). In Ashkenazi Jews, 95% of patients but only 40% of unaffected controls are HLA-DR4. DR4 is also strongly associated with PV in non-Ashkenazi Jews and in Caucasians, but an additional strong association with DRw6 is also observed (Szafer et al., 1987). Overall, more than 95% of PV patients possess either DR4 or DRw6.

Almost all PV patients have the DR4 subtype Dw10, a specificity which is common in Jews but infrequent in Caucasians (Amar et al., 1984; Scharf et al., 1988b). Comparison of DR and DQ allelic sequences reveals that Dw10 differs from the other DR4 subtypes in its DRβ1 chain as discussed above. This suggests that the Dw10 DRβ1 third HVR might be responsible for susceptibility to PV in all ethnic groups. Moreover, one of two known DRw6 DRB1 alleles is identical in its third HVR to that of DR4/Dw10. Scharf et al. (1988a) found this DRB1 sequence in 90% of DR4-positive PV patients but in only 36% of DR4-positive controls. However, although this sequence is also seen in DRw6 haplotypes, in this study it was only present in 25% of DRw6-positive patients. Thus DR4-associated but not DRw6-associated susceptibility may be explained by a sequence motif in the third HVR.

Ahmed et al. (1990) reported that 75% of Jewish PV patients have at least one of two distinct extended haplotypes, both of which include DR4/DQw8. In non-Jewish patients from Europe and North America both DR4/DQw8 and DRw6/DQw5 haplotypes were seen with equal frequency, and the extended haplotypes common in Jewish patients were exceptional. The authors concluded that there are two separate PV susceptibility alleles, one arising on a DR4/DQw8 haplotype in Ashkenazi Jews and another arising more recently on a DRw6/DQw5 haplotype in southern Europe (Ahmed et al., 1991).

Recent studies have suggested that susceptibility maps closely to DQ. By analysing all the polymorphic loci (DRB1, DRB3, DQA1, DQB1 and DPB1) on DRw6 haplotypes in PV patients and controls, the same authors have been able to demonstrate that DRw6-associated susceptibility is conferred by an allele of DQB1 (called DQB1.3) (Scharf et al., 1989). It is of some interest that this allele differs from the more common allele DQB1.1, which is not associated with susceptibility, by a single amino-acid substitution at position 57, the same residue implicated in susceptiblity to IDDM. By oligonucleotide dot-blot analysis, this DQB1 allele was then found in 100% of DRw6-positive Jewish PV patients but in less than 7% of matched controls (Sinha et al., 1988).

Multiple sclerosis

Multiple sclerosis is a disease of the central nervous system characterized by multiple episodes of inflammation and demyelination. Plasma cells are present within MS plaques, and also appear in normal looking white matter in more advanced cases (Adams, 1983). The persistence of small numbers of plasma cells may explain the presence, and continual synthesis, of oligoclonal IgG in the CSF. In addition to B-cells, T-cells and macrophages are found in the initial acute lesions (Traugott et al., 1983). There is a corresponding increase in the number of cells seen in the CSF during the acute phase of MS, and this rise comprises mainly T-cells. Phenotypic analysis of these cells shows an increased ratio of $CD4^+$ to $CD8^+$ cells. Activated lymphocytes ($IL-2R^+$) are found in perivascular areas of the brain in some patients with MS (Woodroofe et al., 1986). No target antigen has been identified in MS. However, experimental allergic encephalomyelitis (EAE), which resembles MS in many ways, can be produced in animals by immunization with myelin, major basic protein (MBP) or MBP fragments, as discussed in Chapter 5.

Population studies

The first reports of an association between MS and the HLA system were published in 1972 (Bertrams et al., 1972; Naito et al., 1972), and it was soon established that there was a reproducible association with HLA-A3 and -B7. Shortly afterwards, a more significant association with an HLA-D locus product was discovered (Jersild et al., 1973), later identified as DR2/Dw2 and present in 40–70% of MS patients (Fog et al., 1977; Thorsby et al., 1977). MS is a disease of Caucasians, especially races of northern European extraction; it is rare in Japanese and blacks, and virtually unheard of in Eskimos and Bantu. The DR2 association is strongest in northern Europe, and is also observed in migrant populations in North America and Australasia which originated in northern Europe.

Serological studies indicate that DR2 is not itself a susceptibility gene for MS. For instance there is no significant DR2 association in patients from the Orkney Islands (Poskanzer et al., 1980), despite this region having the highest prevalence of MS yet described. Secondly, MS is extremely rare in Hungarian gypsies, despite there being a high frequency of DR2 in this population (Gyodi et al., 1981). Although the predominant association is with DR2, associations with DR4 have been reported in southern Italy (Compston, 1978), Sardinia (Marrosu et al., 1988), and Jordan (Kurdi et al., 1977). No consistent association has been reported in Israel or Japan. In a serological study of Scottish patients, it was found that DQw1 was more strongly associated with MS than was DR2 (Francis et al., 1987b).

Family studies

From a population-based sample of 611 patients, Ebers identified 40 sibling pairs, and found that the rate of haplotype sharing did not differ from that expected (Ebers et al., 1982). Also in a population-based study, Govaerts et al. (1985) analysed extended haplotype sharing in 155 patients. Although the expected weak association between MS and DR2 was present, there was no haplotype or allelic recombination significantly linked to disease. Twenty sib-pairs and two trios of MS were also studied, but again there was no distortion of the random distribution of haplotypes. However, Francis et al. (1987a) have shown that the extended haplotype HLA-B7, C4B*3, C4B*1, Bf*S, DR2, DQw1 accounted for 18.9% and 24.2% of parental haplotypes from multiplex and single case families, respectively, in contrast to only 2.3% of parental haplotypes from control families ($P < 0.05$, $P < 0.01$). These data indicate strongly that the HLA region contributes to susceptibility to MS.

Molecular studies

Several analyses of class II RFLPs in MS have been published, confirming the association of MS with DR2,Dw2,DQw6 (Cohen et al., 1984; Marcadet et al., 1985; Jacobson et al., 1986; Serjeantson et al., 1986; Semana et al., 1988; Gogolin et al., 1989). Several of these studies have shown the strongest association with DQB1 restriction fragments, suggesting that susceptibility maps more closely to DQ than to DR. Recently, in a study of 45 Swedish MS patients and 166 Danish controls, a significant association with DPw4, which is independent of DR2, has been described by allogenotyping with DPA1 and DPB1 probes (Ødum et al., 1988). It has not proved possible to identify critical shared stretches of sequence for MS in the same way it has in the case of IDDM, RA, and PV. This possibility was suggested by Vartdal et al. (1989) who demonstrated extensive regions of shared sequence in the DQB1 genes of DR2, DR4, and DRw6 haplotypes in Norwegian MS patients (amino-acid residues 10–29, 31–52, 58–69 and 71–83). However, this has not been clearly seen in other populations of MS patients. Nor is the concept of a disease-specific allele tenable in that the N-terminal domain sequences of DRB1, DQA1 and DQB1 genes were determined in four MS patients, and proved to be identical to those found commonly in healthy individuals.

Evidence that transcomplementation may contribute to susceptibility to MS has come from a RFLP analysis of subjects from Northern Ireland and northeast Scotland (Heard et al., 1989). A cluster of DQA1 restriction fragments exhibiting an allelic relationship to DR2,DQw6 was increased in MS patients independently of DR2, and moreover, the relative risk of possessing both a DR2 haplotype and this RFLP cluster was 11.3. The cluster correlated closely with DR7 and DRw8 haplotypes, raising the possibility of transcomplementation between genes on these haplotypes. These findings could not be confirmed in a lower prevalence population (southern England), further implying that the true susceptibility gene(s) for MS remain to be identified (Francis et al., 1991).

Most patients with MS have a disease course characterized by relapses and remissions (R/R MS). Many will, however, eventually enter a secondary phase in which their symptoms evolve progressively. Between 9% and 37% of patients have an illness which is progressive from onset (primarily chronic progressive, PCP MS), and it is possible that R/R MS and PCP MS may be separate disease entities. However, efforts to differentiate between these two forms of the disease by serological HLA class II typing have yielded inconclusive results. Recently, Olerup et al. (1987, 1989) have reported a strong correlation between R/R and PCP MS and DQB1 restriction fragment polymorphisms. A TaqI DQB1 RF pattern seen in DR4/DQw8, DR7/DQw9, and DRw8/DQw4 haplotypes was found in 65% of PCP MS and only 27% of R/R MS ($P < 0.001$).

A DQB1 allelic pattern seen in DR3-DRw17/DQw2 haplotypes was found in 32% of R/R MS and only 4% of PCP MS ($P < 0.005$). These data indicating immuno-genetic heterogeneity between two clinical forms of MS support the idea that MS may be aetiologically heterogeneous.

Coeliac disease

Coeliac disease (CD) is an inflammatory disease of the jejunal mucosa which is caused by abnormal sensitivity to α-gliadin present in dietary gluten. Susceptibility to gluten sensitivity is genetically determined, at least some of it being encoded in the MHC. There is a 70% concordance rate between monozygotic twins with CD and 10–15% concordance among other first-degree relatives. Strong associations with the sero-logically defined haplotypes DR3,DQw2 and DR7,DQw2 have been found in most populations studied (Ek et al., 1978; DeMarchi et al., 1979). Several of these studies have established that risk is increased particularly in DR3/DR7 (and in Latin populations with DR5/DR7), a situation analogous to that seen in IDDM (Scholz and Albert, 1983; Tiwari et al., 1984). In some studies DR2 is negatively associated with CD and thus may be protective. RFLP studies of the DQ region genes in CD have indicated a strong association with DQA1. Roep et al. (1988) found a 4.0 kb BglII DQA1 restriction fragment in 97% of CD patients and in 56% of controls (relative risk 14.9) and subsequently showed that at the protein level a DQa chain associated with this fragment was present in 100% of CD patients studied. There is also evidence that transcomplementation involving DQα and β chains might be a contributory mechanism to CD susceptibility. While the highest individual risk of CD is conferred by the DR3,DQw2 haplotype, DR7 in association with DR3 or DR5 increases the risk further. The (DR3,)DQw2α chain sequence is identical to that of (DR5,)DQw7α while (DR3,)DQw2β differs from (DR7,)DQw2β at only a single position (Karr et al., 1986). Thus DR5,DQw7/DR7,DQw2 heterozygotes could, by transcomplementation, express the same, or almost the same, DQαβ heterodimers formed by DQA1 and DQB1 genes in *cis* position on the DR3,DQw2 haplotype (Sollid et al., 1989).

However, it has become evident that products of the HLA-DP loci also play a prominant part in susceptibility to CD. The role of DP in autoimmune diseases have been studied less frequently than DR and DQ due to the complexity of the primed lymphocyte typing method, but has recently become more accessible with the advent of RFLP and other molecular techniques. Two allelic variants of DPA1 and 14 alleles of DPB1 can be distinguished by sequence analysis, with most of the variability in DPB1 being clustered in hypervariable regions similar to DQB1 (Bugawan et al., 1988). A RsaI DPB1 restriction fragment is significantly increased in both Caucasian and Latin-American CD patients (Herrera et al., 1989). Sequence analysis of Class II genes associated with the CD DR3 haplotype shows that all DP, DQ and DR alleles were identical to those which are also seen in healthy subjects, but probing of PCR-amplified DNA with allele-specific probes has demonstrated a significant increase in the frequencies of DPB1.1 and DPB1.3, both of which are related to the RsaI restriction fragment (Kagnoff et al., 1989). Moreover the association of DPB1 alleles with CD seems to be independent of linkage to DR3 and DR7, indicating that risk may be increased particularly in individuals possessing specific combinations of DP and DQ alleles (Howell et al., 1988; Bugawan et al., 1989). The joint segregation in CD patients of these DP alleles with those encoding the specificities DR3 and DQw2 indicates that the extended haplotype conferring susceptibility to CD encompasses the entire HLA-D region. A relatively simple mechanism to explain these data would be that mixed isotype αβ pairing (e.g. DRα/DQβ) is responsible for T-cell activation (see below). However, it is also possible that the products of other, as yet unidentified, loci in the HLA region are also involved (Rosenberg et al., 1989; Sargent et al., 1989).

Ankylosing spondylitis

Ankylosing spondylitis (AS) is an inflammatory disease, and the most important of a spectrum of seronegative spondyloarthropathies. The disease affects principally the joints of the spine and pelvis, but other joints may also be involved and systemic manifestations are sometimes seen. AS differs from the autoimmune diseases discussed previously in several ways, including: (1) the strength of its association with HLA; (2) its primary association with a class I rather than a class II allele; and (3) its relationship to a known infectious agent. Evidence from many sources has led to the hypothesis that AS is the result of repeated episodes of *Klebsiella*-reactive arthritis in HLA-B27 positive subjects.

The B27 association

The dramatic association between B27 and AS was first reported in 1973 by Schlosstein et al. (1973) and Brewerton et al. (1973). B27 was present in up to 96%

of patients as opposed to only 4–8% of controls, and these findings have since been confirmed in many later studies in several different ethnic groups (see Tiwari and Terasaki, 1985, pp. 85–100). However, only a very small proportion of B27-positive individuals develop AS implying that the presence of AS is, in most cases, necessary but not sufficient to cause AS. The frequency of B27 in AS patients is in fact sufficiently high to make it possible that it plays a direct aetiological role in the development of the disease. Where racial differences are observed, they tend to highlight the importance of B27. For instance, although B27 is uncommon in Japanese, its frequency in AS patients is as high as in Caucasians. AS and B27 are both unknown in Australian aborigines. AS is much less common in females than in males, but its association with B27 is just as strong (Levitin et al., 1976). AS is weakly associated with HLA-Cw1 and Cw2, but this is due to linkage disequilibrium between this locus and B27 (van den Berg-Loonen et al., 1977).

However, family studies suggest that susceptibility to AS is more complex than simply the effect of a dominant HLA gene. There have been several pedigree analyses in which AS fails to segregate completely with B27, indicating that other loci may also be involved. In support of this is the recent observation that the presence of Bw60 increases the risk of AS in B27-positive subjects by a factor of three (Robinson et al., 1989b). The development of AS in B27-negative subjects would appear at first glance to argue against a direct pathogenetic role for B27 and may suggest that B27 is merely a closely linked marker of another causative gene. The case for this explanation is strengthened by the recent discovery of a number of previously unknown loci centromeric to, and closely linked to, HLA-B (Spies et al., 1989) (see Chapter 9). However, disease heterogeneity can provide a more likely explanation for B27-negative AS; there is considerable clinical overlap between AS and the other seronegative arthropathies and no definitive diagnostic test exists for any of them. There is limited evidence that homozygosity for B27 further increases the risk. Strikingly, no significant association with any class II alleles has been described.

Cross-reactivity between B27 and Klebsiella

In 1979 two groups reported independently that anti-B27 antisera reacted against *Klebsiella* and some other enterobacteria, and that anti-*Klebsiella* antibodies lysed lymphocytes from B27-positive AS patients (Ebringer, 1979; Seager et al., 1979; Geczy and Yap, 1979). More recently it has been shown that anti-B27 monoclonal antibodies cross-react with antigens found on *Klebsiella*, *Salmonella*, *Shigella* and *Yersinia*. All of these bacteria are associated with reactive arthritis in B27-positive individuals, but only *Klebsiella* can be isolated from the faeces of patients with AS (reviewed by Ebringer, 1989). At least six variants of B27 have been identified by means of sequence analysis. By performing a computerized homology search it was found that two of these variants, B27 and B27.1, share a hexamer peptide sequence QTDRED with *Klebsiella pneumoniae* nitrogenase (Chen et al., 1987; Schwimmbeck et al., 1987). This has led to speculation that AS is the result of molecular mimicry causing the initiation of a humoral autoimmune process. However, a number of observations remain unexplained by this hypothesis which consequently has failed to gain universal acceptance. Firstly, since HLA class I molecules have a widespread tissue distribution, the preference of the disease process for certain synovial joints cannot be accounted for. Secondly, in one recent study, antibodies against the shared hexamer were found with equal frequencies in AS patients and controls (Tsuchiya et al., 1989). Thirdly, it is now known that B27 is polymorphic, and that AS is associated with all of the B27 subtypes, thus it would be necessary to postulate a group of structural similarities between bacteria and each of the B27 subtypes. It is clear that further study is required to elucidate the mechanisms whereby potentially cross-reactive determinants might initiate a class I-associated autoimmune response.

B27 and autoimmunity

Recent studies have revealed the structure of the B27 subtypes and shed light on how they might be involved in an autoimmune process as a T-cell restriction element rather than as an autoantigen. Seven subtypes of B27 have been identified and sequenced (Lopez de Castro, 1989; Choo and Hansen, 1989) and their three-dimensional structure can be predicted from that of HLA-A2 (Bjorkman et al., 1987). AS appears to be associated equally with all subtypes of B27, except perhaps B2703, and this implies that susceptibility is a function of conserved rather than variable sequence motifs within the molecule. Furthermore, B27 differs from other class I molecules most markedly in the region of the antigen-binding groove, hinting strongly that disease susceptibility is related to the peptide-binding function of the molecule.

The individual B27 subtypes themselves show considerable polymorphism in the region of the antigen-binding groove, but Benjamin and Parham (1990) have shown that there is a motif of six residues (His-9, Glu-45, Cys-67, Lys-70, Ala-71, Gln-97) which is unique to B27, and is conserved in all of the subtypes. These conserved residues lie in close proximity to each other near the mouth of the 45 pocket (Garrett et al., 1989). Thus the pocket of B27 has a unique structure and moreover is conserved between its various subtypes. In this way all the subtypes would share the same ability to present a peptide to cytotoxic T-cells (CTL) in a manner which is peculiar to B27. This hypothesis proposes that T-cells are sensitized initially by exposure to a foreign peptide (from *Klebsiella* for instance) and subsequently become responsive to an autologous peptide fragment derived from synovial tissue and which is presented to the CTL by B27. Taurog and El-Zaatari (1988) have also drawn attention to the unpaired cysteine residue at position 67 of the B27 molecule. This points in towards the antigen-binding groove and has the potential to form a strong disulphide bond with a thiol group present on a peptide fragment within the groove. Mutagenesis experiments have shown that changing the amino acid at position 67 can have a major effect on the conformation of the groove, and by inference probably exerts a profound influence over its ability to bind antigenic peptides. This argument has been adapted by Benjamin and Parham (1990) who have argued that the conformation and function of the antigen-binding groove is likely to be altered by a thiol group binding to Cys-67. If the thiol-containing peptide was derived from synovial tissues, and the redox/pH conditions necessary for formation of the disulphide linkage only existed in certain joints, then this model might be capable of explaining the tissue specificity seen in AS.

The future

As discussed in Chapter 3, an autoimmune CD4+ T-cell response requires the recognition by the T-cell receptor of a self peptide within the antigen-binding cleft of a self class II molecule. Detailed structural and functional analysis of each of these is necessary for an effective understanding of the processes resulting in the breakdown of self-tolerance, which in turn might allow the development of strategies to block these processes in a highly specific fashion. It has been known for some time that some experimental models of autoimmune disease can be suppressed with anti-class II monoclonal antibodies (mAb) (Offner et al., 1986). More recently, it has been shown that there is extremely limited $V\beta$ gene usage by T-cells in EAE, and that the disease can be prevented with anti-$(V\beta 8.2)$ T-cell receptor mAb (Acha-Orbea et al., 1988; Zamvil et al., 1988; Urban et al., 1988; Owhashi and Heber-Katz, 1988). Recently, restricted TcR Va gene rearrangements have also been found in affected brain tissue of MS patients (Oksenberg et al., 1990), increasing the hope that it will become possible to treat this condition with specific forms of immunotherapy. Another approach has been to treat an animal with a synthetic peptide designed so as to have an extremely high affinity for the antigen-binding cleft of a class II susceptibility allele (Wraith et al., 1989). Such a peptide would successfully compete with a self-peptide and thus block the MHC–TcR interaction. In theory at least, an effective immunotherapy could therefore be devised without it ever being necessary to identify the autoantigen against which the disease process is being directed. If such therapies can be devised, they offer the prospect of effective treatment for the whole spectrum of human autoimmune disease.

References

Acha-Orbea H., Mitchell, D.J., Timmerman, L. et al. (1988). Limited heterogeneity of T cell receptors from lymphocytes mediating autoimmune encephalomyelitis allows specific immune intervention. *Cell* **54**: 263–273.

Adams, C.W.M. (1983). *Multiple Sclerosis* (eds C.W.M. Adams, J.F. Hallpike and W.W. Tourtellotte), pp. 203–240. Chapman & Hall, London.

Adams, D.D. (1958). The presence of an abnormal thyroid-stimulating hormone in the serum of some thyrotoxic patients. *J. Clin. Endocrinol. Metab.* **18**: 699–712.

Ahmed, A.R. (1980). Pemphigus: current concepts. *Ann. Intern. Med.* **92**: 396–405.

Ahmed, A.R., Yunis, E.J., Khatri, K. et al. (1990). Major histocompatibility complex haplotype studies in Ashkenazi Jewish patients with pemphigus vulgaris. *Proc. Natl Acad. Sci. USA* **87**: 7658–7662.

Ahmed, A.R., Wagner, R., Khatri, K. et al. (1991). Major histocompatibility complex haplotypes and class II genes in non-Jewish patients with pemphigus vulgaris. *Proc. Natl Acad. Sci. USA* **88**: 5056–5060.

Amar, A., Rubinstein, N., Hachem-Zadeh, S. et al. (1984). Is predisposition to pemphigus vulgaris in Jewish patients mediated by HLA-Dw10 and DR4? *Tissue Antigens* **23**: 17–22.

Amiel, J.L. (1967). *Histocompatibility Testing 1967* (eds E.S. Curtoni, P.L. Mattiuz and R.M. Tosi), pp. 79–81, Munksgaard, Copenhagen.

Aparicio, J.M.R., Wakisaka, A., Tokada, A. et al. (1988). HLA-DQ system and insulin dependent diabetes mellitus in Japanese: does it contribute to the development of IDDM as it does in Caucasians? *Immunogenetics* **28**: 240–246.

Atar, D., Dyrberg, T., Michelsen, B. et al. (1989). Site-specific antibodies distinguish single amino acid substitutions in position 57 in HLA-DQ β-chain alleles associated with insulin-dependent diabetes. *J. Immunol.* **143**: 533–538.

Bach, F.H., Rich, S.S., Barbosa, J. et al. (1985). Insulin-dependent diabetes-associated HLA-D region encoded determinants. *Human Immunol.* **12**: 59–64.

Begovich, A.B., Bugawan, T.L., Nepom, B.S. et al. (1989). A specific DPβ allele is associated with pauciarticular juvenile rheumatoid arthritis but not adult rheumatoid arthritis. *Proc. Natl Acad. Sci. USA* **86**: 9489–9493.

Benjamin, R. and Parham, P. (1990). Guilt by association: HLA-B27 and ankylosing spondylitis. *Immunol. Today* **11**: 137–142.

Bertrams, J.K., Kuwert, E. and Liedtke, U. (1972). HL-A antigens and multiple sclerosis. *Tissue Antigens* **2**: 405–408.

Bill, J., Appel, V.B. and Palmer, E. (1988). An analysis of T cell receptor variable region gene expression in major histocompatibility complex disparate mice. *Proc. Natl Acad. Sci. USA* **85**: 9184–9188.

Bjorkman, P.J., Saper, M.A., Samraoui, B. et al. (1987). Structure of the human class I histocompatibility antigen, HLA-A2. *Nature* **329**: 506–512.

Bottazzo, G.F., Dean, B.M., McNally, J.M. et al. (1985). In situ characterisation of autoimmune phenomena and expression of HLA molecules in the pancreas of diabetic insulitis. *N. Engl. J. Med.* **313**: 353–360.

Brewerton, D.A., Caffrey, M., Hart, F.D. et al. (1973). Ankylosing spondylitis and HL-A27. *Lancet* **1**: 904–907.

Bugawan, T.L., Horn, G.T., Long, C.M. et al. (1988). Analysis of HLA-DP allelic sequence polymorphism using the in vitro enzymatic DNA amplification of DP alpha and DP beta loci. *J. Immunol.* **141**: 4024–4030.

Bugawan, T.L., Angelini, G., Larrick, J. et al. (1989). A combination of a particular HLA-DP β allele and an HLA-DQ heterodimer confers susceptibility to coeliac disease. *Nature* **339**: 470–473.

Campbell, I.L. and Harrison, L.C. (1990). Molecular pathology of type 1 diabetes. *Mol. Biol. Med.* **7**: 299–309.

Carrier, C., Mollen, N., Ginsberg-Fellner, F. et al. (1989). DQA1 restriction fragment length polymorphisms and insulin dependent diabetes mellitus: a BglII fragment labels a subset of B8,DR3 haplotypes uniquely associated with insulin dependent diabetes mellitus. *Hum. Immunol.* **26**: 344–352.

Chen, J.H., Kono, D.H., Yong, Z. et al. (1987). A Yersinia pseudotuberculosis protein which cross-reacts with HLA-B27. *J. Immunol.* **13**: 3003–3011.

Choo, S.Y. and Hansen, J.A. (1989). *Human Immunology, Program and Abstracts*. 15th Annual ASHI Meeting, abstract 4.2–02, Elsevier, Amsterdam.

Christiansen, F.T., Saueracker, G.C., Leaver, A.L. et al. (1990). Characterization of MHC ancestral haplotypes associated with insulin-dependent diabetes mellitus: evidence for involvement of non-HLA genes. *J. Immunogenet.* **17**: 379–386.

Clarkson, R., Bate, A.S., Grennan, D.M. et al. (1990). DQw7 and the C4B null allele in rheumatoid arthritis and Felty's syndrome. *Ann. Rheum. Dis.* **49**: 976–979.

Cohen, D., Cohen, O., Marcadet, A. et al. (1984). Class II HLA-DC β-chain DNA restriction fragments differentiate among HLA-DR2 individuals in insulin-dependent diabetes and multiple sclerosis. *Proc. Natl Acad. Sci. USA* **81**: 1774–1778.

Cohen-Haguenauer, O., Robbins, E., Massart, C. et al. (1985). A systematic study of the HLA class IIb DNA restriction fragments in insulin dependent diabetes mellitus. *Proc. Natl Acad. Sci. USA* **83**: 3335–3339.

Compston, D.A.S. (1978). HLA and neurologic disease. *Neurology* **28**: 413–414.

Cowan, E.P., Pierce, M.L., McFarland, H.F. et al. (1991). HLA-DR and -DQ allelic sequences in multiple sclerosis patients are identical to those found in the general population. *Hum. Immunol.* **32**: 203–210.

DeMarchi, M., Borelli, I., Olivetti, E. et al. (1979). Two HLA-D and DR alleles are associated with coeliac disease. *Tissue Antigens* **14**: 309–316.

Deschamps, I., Lestradet, H., Bonaiti, C. et al. (1980). HLA gentotype studies in juvenile insulin-dependent diabetes. *Diabetologia* **19**: 189–193.

Deschamps, I., Marcelli-Barge, A., Lallemand, N. et al. (1988). Study of cis and trans interactions between extended HLA-haplotypes in insulin-dependent diabetes. *Tissue Antigens* **31**: 259–269.

DuPont, B. (1989). *Immunobiology of HLA*. Springer-Verlag, New York.

Duquesnoy, R.J., Marrari, M., Hackbarth, S. et al. (1984). Serological and cellular definition of a new HLA-DR associated determinant, MC1, and its association with rheumatoid arthritis. *Hum. Immunol.* **10**: 165–176.

Ebers, G.C., Paty, D.W., Stiller, C.R. et al. (1982). HLA typing in multiple sclerosis sibling pairs. *Lancet* **1**: 88–90.

Ebringer, A. (1979). Ankylosing spondylitis, immune-response-genes and molecular mimicry. *Lancet* **1**: 1186 (letter).

Ebringer, A. (1989). The relationship between Klebsiella infection and ankylosing spondylitis. *Bailliere's Clin. Rheumatol.* **3**: 321–338.

Ek, J., Albrechtsen, D., Solheim, B.G. et al. (1978). Strong association between the HLA-Dw3-related B cell alloantigen-DRw3 and coeliac disease. *Scand. J. Gastroenterol.* **13**: 229–233.

Festenstein, H., Awad, J., Hitman, G.A. et al. (1986). New HLA DNA polymorphisms associated with autoimmune diseases. *Nature* **322**: 64–67.

Fink, C.W. and Stastny, P. (1980). Results of serologic HLA-DR typing in juvenile arthritis and adult rheumatoid arthritis. *Arthritis and Rheumat.* **23**: 673 (abstract).

Fog, T., Schuller, E., Jersild, C. et al. (1977). *HLA and Disease* (ed. J. Dausset and A. Svejgaard), pp. 108–125. Munksgaard, Copenhagen.

Francis, D.A., Batchelor, J.R., McDonald, W.I. et al. (1987a). HLA genetic determinants in familial MS: a study from the Grampian Region of Scotland. *Tissue Antigens* **29**: 7–12.

Francis, D.A., Batchelor, J.R., McDonald, W.I. et al. (1987b). Multiple sclerosis in north-east Scotland: an association with HLA-DQw1. *Brain* **110**: 181–196.

Francis, D.A., Thompson, A.J., Brookes, P. et al. (1991). Multiple sclerosis and HLA: is the susceptibility gene really HLA-DR or -DQ? *Hum. Immunol.* **32**: 119–124.

Garrett, T.P.J., Saper, M.A., Bjorkman, P.J. et al. (1989). Specificity pockets for the side chains of peptide antigens in HLA-Aw68. *Nature* **342**: 692–696.

Geczy, A.F. and Yap, J. (1979). HLA-B27, Klebsiella and ankylosing spondylitis. *Lancet* **1**: 719–720 (letter).

Glass, D., Litvin, D., Wallace, K. et al. (1980). Early-onset pauciarticular juvenile rheumatoid arthritis associated with human leukocyte antigen-DRw5, iritis, and antinuclear antibody. *J. Clin. Invest.* **66**: 426–429.

Gogolin, K.J., Kolaga, V.J., Baker, L. et al. (1989). Subtypes of HLA-DQ and -DR defined by DQB1 RFLPs: allele frequencies in the general population and in insulin dependent diabetes (IDDM) and multiple sclerosis patients. *Ann. Hum. Genet.* **53**: 327–338.

Goronzy, J., Weyand, C.M. and Fathman, C.G. (1986). Shared T cell recognition sites on human histocompatibility leukocyte antigen class II molecules of patients with seropositive rheumatoid arthritis. *J. Clin. Invest.* **77**: 1042–1049.

Govaerts, A., Gony, J., Martin-Mondière, C. et al. (1985). HLA and multiple sclerosis: population and families study. *Tissue Antigens* **25**: 187–199.

Gran, J.T., Husby, G. and Thorsby, E. (1983). HLA DR antigens and gold toxicity. *Ann. Rheum. Dis.* **42**: 63–66.

Gregersen, P.K., Moriuchi, T., Karr, R.W. et al. (1986). Polmorphism of HLA-DR β chains in DR4, – 7, and -9 haplotypes: implications for the mechanisms of allelic variation. *Proc. Natl Acad. Sci. USA* **83**: 9149–9153.

Gregersen, P.K., Silver, J. and Winchester, R.J. (1987). The shared epitope hypothesis. An approach to understanding the molecular genetics of susceptibility to rheumatoid arthritis. *Arthritis Rheum.* **30**: 1205–1213.

Grennan, D.M. and Sanders, P.A. (1988). Rheumatoid arthritis. *Bailliere's Clin. Rheumatol.* **2**: 585–601.

Gyodi, E., Tauszik, T., Petranyi, G. et al. (1981). The HLA antigen distribution in the gypsy population in Hungary. *Tissue Antigens* **18**: 1–12.

Hammond, S.R., McLeod, J.G., Millingen, K.S. et al. (1988). The epidemiology of multiple sclerosis in three Australian cities: Perth, Newcastle and Hobart. *Brain* **111**: 1–25.

Herrera, M., Chertkoff, L., Palavecino, E. et al. (1989). Restriction fragment length polymorphism in HLA class II genes of Latin-American caucasian celiac disease patients. *Hum. Immunol.* **26**: 272–280.

Hillarby, M.C., Clarkson, R., Grennan, D.M. et al. (1991). Immunogenetic heterogeneity in rheumatoid disease as illustrated by different MHC associations (DQ, Dw, and C4) in articular and extra-articular subsets. *Br. J. Rheumatol.* **30**: 5–9.

Hohlfeld, R., Conti-Tronconi, B., Kalies, I. et al. (1985). Genetic restriction of autoreactive acetyl choline receptor-specific T lymphocytes in myasthenia gravis. *J. Immunol.* **135**: 2393–2399.

Horn, G.T., Bugawan, T.L., Long, C.M. et al. (1988). Allelic sequence variation of the HLA-DQ loci: relationship to serology and to insulin-dependent diabetes susceptibility. *Proc. Natl Acad. Sci. USA* **85**: 6012–6016.

Howell, M.D., Smith, J.R., Austin, R.K. et al. (1988). An extended HLA-D region haplotype associated with celiac disease. *Proc. Natl Acad. Sci. USA* **85**: 222–226.

Hyer, R.N., Julier, C., Buckley, J.D. et al. (1991). High-resolution linkage mapping for susceptibility genes in human polygenic disease: insulin dependent diabetes mellitus and chromosome 11q. *Am. J. Hum. Genet.* **48**: 243–257.

Ilonen, J., Herva, E., Tiilikainen, A. et al. (1978). HLA-Dw2 as a marker of resistance against juvenile diabetes mellitus. *Tissue Antigens* **11**: 144–146.

Jacobson, S., Sorrentino, R., Nepom, G.T. et al. (1986). DNA restriction fragment length polymorphism of HLA-DR2: correlation with HLA-DR2 associated functions. *J. Neuroimmunol.* **12**: 195–203.

Jersild, C., Fog, T., Hansen, G.S. et al. (1973). Histocompatibility determinants in multiple sclerosis with special reference to clinical course. *Lancet* **2**: 1221–1225.

Juji, T., Satake, M., Honda, Y. et al. (1984). HLA antigens in Japanese patients with narcolepsy. *Tissue Antigens* **24**: 316–319.

Kagnoff, M.F., Harwood, J.I., Bugawan, T.L. et al. (1989). Structural analysis of the HLA-DR, -DQ, and -DP alleles on the celiac disease-associated HLA-DR3 (DRw17) haplotype. *Proc. Natl Acad. Sci. USA* **86**: 6274–6278.

Kappler, J., Kotzin, B., Herron, L. et al. (1989). Vβ-specific stimulation of human T cells by staphylococcal toxins. *Science* **244**: 811–813.

Karr, R.W., Gregersen, P.K., Obata, F. et al. (1986). Analysis of DRβ and DQβ chain cDNA clones from the DR7 haplotype. *J. Immunol.* **137**: 2886–2893.

Khan, M.A., Kushner, I., Ballou, S.P. et al. (1979). Familial rheumatoid arthritis and HLA-DRW4. *Lancet* **1**: 921–922.

Koide, Y. and Yoshida, T.O. (1990). The unique nucleotide sequence of the A beta gene in the NOD mouse is shared with its nondiabetic sister strains, the ILI and the CTS mouse. *Int. Immunol.* **2**: 189–192.

Kurdi, A., Ayesh, I., Abdallat, A. et al. (1977). Different B-lymphocyte alloantigens associated with multiple sclerosis in Arabs and North Europeans. *Lancet* **1**: 1123–1125.

Kurtzke, J.F. (1980). Epidemiologic contributions to multiple sclerosis: an overview. *Neurology* **30**: 61–79.

Lanchbury, J.S., Sakkas, L.I., Marsh, S.G. et al. (1989). HLA-DQ β 3.1 allele is a determinant of susceptibility to DR4-associated rheumatoid arthritis. *Hum. Immunol.* **26**: 59–71.

Lang, B., Melchers, I., Urlacher, A. et al. (1990). HLA-DR1 and DRw6 association in DR4-negative rheumatoid arthritis patients. *Rheumatol. Int.* **10**: 171–175.

Levitin, P.M., Gough, W.W., and Davis, J.S. (1976). HLA-B27 antigen in women with ankylosing spondylitis. *JAMA* **235**: 2621–2622.

Lopez de Castro, J.A. (1989). HLA-B27 and HLA-A2 subtypes: structure, evolution and function. *Immunol. Today* **10**: 239–246.

Lundin, K.E., Gaudernack, G., Qvigstad, E. et al. (1988). T lymphocyte clones recognizing an HLA-DQw3.2-associated epitope involving residue 57 on the DQ β chain. *Hum. Immunol.* **22**: 235–246.

Lundin, K.E., Rønningen, K.S., Spurkland, A. et al. (1989). HLA-DQ antigens and DQ β amino acid 57 of Japanese patients with insulin-dependent diabetes mellitus: detection of a DRw8DQw8 haplotype. *Tissue Antigens* **34**: 233–241.

Marcadet, A., Massart, C., Semana, G. et al. (1985). Association of class II HLA-DQβ chain DNA restriction fragments with multiple sclerosis. *Immunogenetics* **22**: 93–96.

Marrosu, M.G., Muntoni, F., Murru, M.R. et al. (1988). Sardinian multiple sclerosis is associated wth HLA-DR4: a serologic and molecular analysis. *Neurology* **38**: 1749–1753.

Matthews, W.B. (1985). *McAlpine's Multiple Sclerosis* (eds W.B. Matthews, J.R. Batchelor, E.D. Acheson, and R.O. Weller). pp. 49–72. Churchill Livingstone, Edinburgh.

McDevitt, H.O. and Benacerraf, B. (1969). Genetic control of specific immune responses. *Adv. Immunol.* **11**: 31–55.

McInerney, M.F., Rath, S., and Janeway, C.A. (1991). Exclusive expression of MHC class II proteins on CD45+ cells in pancreatic islet cells of NOD mice. *Diabetes* **40**: 648–651.

Melin-Aldana, H., Giannini, E.H., and Glass, D.N. (1990). Immunogenetics of early onset pauciarticular juvenile rheumatoid arthritis. *J. Rheumatol.* (Suppl.) **26**: 2–6.

Michelson, B. and Lernmark, A. (1987). Molecular cloning of a polymorphic DNA endonuclease fragment associates insulin dependent diabetes mellitus with HLA-DQ. *J. Clin. Invest.* **75**: 1144–1152.

Morel, P.A., Dorman, J.S., Todd, J.A. et al. (1988). Aspartic acid at position 57 of the DQβ chain protects against Type I diabetes: a family study. *Hum. Immunol.* **23**: 126–132.

Morton, N.E., Green, A., Dunsworth, T. et al. (1983). Heterozygous expression of insulin-dependent diabetes mellitus (IDDM) determinants in the HLA system. *Am. J. Hum. Genet.* **35**: 201–213.

Naito, S., Takeshi, T., and Kuroiwa, Y. (1972). Multiple sclerosis: association with HL-A3. *Tissue Antigens* **2**: 1–4.

Nepom, B.S., Palmer, J., Kim, S.J. et al. (1986). Specific genomic markers for the HLA-DQ subregion discriminate between DR4+ insulin-dependent diabetes mellitus and DR4+ seropositive juvenile rheumatoid arthritis. *J. Exp. Med.* **164**: 345–350.

Nepom, B.S., Schwarz, D., Palmer, J.P. et al. (1987). Transcomplementation of HLA genes in IDDM HLA DQ α and β chains produced hybrid molecules in DR3/4 heterozygotes. *Diabetes* **36**: 114–117.

Nepom, G.T., Byers, P., Seyfried, C. et al. (1989). HLA genes associated with rheumatoid arthritis. Identification of susceptibility alleles using specific oligonucleotide probes. *Arthritis Rheum.* **32**: 15–21.

Nerup, J. (1978). HLA studies in diabetes mellitus: A review. *Adv. Metab. Dis.* **9**: 263–277.

Niven, M.J., Hitman, G.A., Pearce, H. et al. (1990). Large haplotype-specific differences in inter-genic distances in human MHC shown by pulsed field electrophoresis mapping of healthy and type 1 diabetic subjects. *Tissue Antigens* **36**: 19–24.

Nunez, G., Moore, S., Ball, G.V. et al. (1980). The inheritance of HLA haplotypes in families with rheumatoid arthritis. *Arthritis Rheum.* **23**: 726–731.

Ødum, N., Hyldig-Nielsen, J.J., Morling, N. et al. (1988). HLA-DP antigens are involved in the susceptibility to multiple sclerosis. *Tissue Antigens* **31**: 235–237.

Oksenberg, J.R., Begovich, A.B., Bell, R.B. et al. (1990). Limited heterogeneity of rearranged T cell receptor Vα transcripts in brains of MS patients. *Nature* **34**: 344–346.

Olerup, O., Fredrikson, S., Olsson, T. et al. (1987). HLA class II genes in chronic progressive and in relapsing/remitting multiple sclerosis *Lancet* **2**: 7507 (letter).

Olerup, O., Hillert, J., Fredrikson, S. et al. (1989). Primarily chronic progressive and relapsing/remitting multiple sclerosis – two immunogenetically distinct disease entities. *Proc. Natl Acad. Sci. USA* **86**: 7113–7118.

Ollier, W., Carthy, D., and Cutbush, S. (1989). HLA-DR4 associated Dw types in rheumatoid arthritis. *Tissue Antigens* **33**: 30–37.

O'Reilly, L.A., Hutchings, P.R., Crocker, P.R. et al. (1991). Characterization of pancreatic islet cell infiltrates in NOD mice: effect of cell transfer and transgene expression. *Eur. J. Immunol.* **21**: 1171–1180.

Owhashi, M. and Heber-Katz, E. (1988). Protection from experimental allergic encephalomyelitis conferred by a monoclonal antibody directed against a shared idiotype on rat T cell receptors specific for myelin basic protein. *J. Exp. Med.* **168**: 2153–2164.

Panayi, G.S., Wooley, P. and Batchelor, J.R. (1978). Genetic basis of rheumatoid disease: HLA antigens, disease manifestations and toxic reactions to drugs. *Br. Med. J.* **2**: 1326–1328.

Pandey, J.P., Goust, J.M., Salier, J.P. et al. (1981). Immunoglobulin G heavy chain (Gm) allotypes in multiple sclerosis. *J. Clin. Invest.* **67**: 1797–1800.

Payami, H., Thomson, G., Khan, M.A. et al. (1986). Genetics of rheumatoid arthritis. *Tissue Antigens* **27**: 57–63.

Poskanzer, D.C., Terasaki, P.I., Prenney, L.B. et al. (1980). Multiple sclerosis in the Orkney and Shetland Islands. III: Histocompatibility determinants. *J. Epidemiol. Community Health* **34**: 253–257.

Robinson, D.M.. Holbeck, S., Palmer, J. et al. (1989a). HLA DQβ3.2 identifies subtypes of DR4+ haplotypes permissive for IDDM. *Genet. Epidemiol.* **6**: 149–154.

Robinson, D.M., van der Linden, S.M., Khan, M.A. et al. (1989b). HLA-Bw60 increases susceptibility to ankylosing spondylitis in HLA-B27+ patients. *Arthritis Rheum.* **32**: 1135–1141.

Roep, B.O., Bontrop, R.E., Peña, A.S. et al. (1988). An HLA-DQα allele identified at DNA and protein level is strongly associated with celiac disease. *Hum. Immunol.* **23**: 271–279.

Ronningen, K.S., Markussen, G., Iwe, T. et al. (1989a). An increased risk of insulin-dependent diabetes mellitus (IDDM) among HLA-DR4,DQw8/DRw8,DQw4 heterozygotes. *Hum. Immunol.* **24**: 165–173.

Ronningen, K.S., Iwe, T., Halstensen, T.S. et al. (1989b). The amino acid at position 57 of the HLA-DQ β chain and susceptibility to develop insulin dependent diabetes mellitus. *Hum. Immunol.* **26**: 215–225.

Rosenberg, W.M., Wordsworth, B.P., Jewell, D.P. et al. (1989). A locus telomeric to HLA-DPB encodes susceptibility to coeliac disease. *Immunogenetics* **30**: 307–310.

Rubinstein, P., Suciu-Foca, N., Nicholson, J.F. et al. (1976). The HLA system in the families of patients with juvenile diabetes mellitus. *J. Exp. Med.* **143**: 1277–1282.

Ryder, L.P., Christy, M., Nerup, J. et al. (1979). HLA studies in diabetics. *Adv. Exp. Med. Biol.* **119**: 41–50.

Sachs, J.A., Cassell, P.G., Festenstein, H. et al. (1987). DQβ restriction fragment length polymorphism and its relationship to insulin dependent diabetes mellitus. *Dis. Markers* **5**: 199–206.

Sargent, C.A., Dunham, I. and Campbell, R.D. (1989). Identification of multiple HTF-island associated genes in the human major histocompatibility complex class III region. *EMBO J.* **8**: 2305–2312.

Scharf, S.J., Friedmann, A., Brautbar, C. et al. (1988a). HLA class II allelic variation and susceptibility to pemphigus vulgaris. *Proc. Natl Acad. Sci. USA* **85**: 3504–3508.

Scharf, S.J., Long, C.M. and Erlich, H.A. (1988b). Sequence analysis of the HLA-DRβ and HLA-DQβ loci from three pemphigus vulgaris patients. *Hum. Immunol.* **22**: 61–69.

Scharf, S.J., Friedmann, A., Steinman, L. et al. (1989). Specific HLA-DQB and HLA-DRB1 alleles confer susceptibility to pemphigus vulgaris. *Proc. Nat Acad. Sci. USA* **86**: 6215–6219.

Schlosstein, L., Terasaki, P.I., Bluestone, J. et al. (1973). High association of a HL-A antigen, w27, with ankylosing spondylitis. *N. Engl. J. Med.* **288**: 704–706.

Scholz, S. and Albert, E. (1983). HLA and diseases: involvement of more than one HLA-linked determinant of disease susceptibility. *Immunol. Rev.* **70**: 77–88.

Schwimmbeck, P.L., Yu, D.T. and Oldstone, M.B. (1987). Autoantibodies to HLA B27 in the sera of HLA B27 patients with ankylosing spondylitis and Reiter's syndrome. Molecular mimicry with *Klebsiella pneumoniae* as potential mechanism of autoimmune disease. *J. Exp. Med.* **166**: 173–181.

Seager, K., Bashir, H.V., Geczy, A.F. et al. (1979). Evidence for a specific B27-associated cell surface marker on lymphocytes of patients with ankylosing spondylitis. *Nature* **277**: 68–70.

Semana, G., Quillivic, F., Madigand, M. et al. (1988). HLA genetic factors involved in familial MS: RFLP study defines a particular DQw1 subtype associated with the disease. In *Trends in European Multiple Sclerosis Research* (eds C. Confraveux, G. Aimard, and M. Devic), Elsevier, Amsterdam.

Serjeantson, S.W., Kohonen-Corish, M.R.J. Dunckley, H. et al. (1986). HLA class II RFLPs are haplotype specific. *Cold Spring Harb. Symp. Quant. Biol.* **51**: 83–89.

Serjeantson, S.W., Ranford, P.R., Kirk, R.L. et al. (1987). HLA-DR and -DQ genotyping in insulin dependent diabetes mellitus in South India. *Dis. Markers* **5**: 101–108.

Sheehy, M.J., Scharf, S.J., Rowe, J.R. et al. (1989). A diabetes-susceptible HLA haplotype is best defined by a combination of HLA-DR and -DQ alleles. *J. Clin. Invest.* **83**: 830–835.

Singh, B., Dillon, T., Fraga, E. et al. (1990). Role of the first external domain of I-A beta chain in immune responses and diabetes in non-obese diabetic (NOD) mice. *J. Autoimmun.* **3**: 507–521.

Sinha, A.A., Brautbar, C., Sfazer, F. et al. (1988). A newly characterized HLA DQβ allele associated with pemphigus vulgaris. *Science* **239**: 1026–1029.

Sollid, L.M., Markussen, G., Ek, J. et al. (1989). Evidence for a primary association of celiac disease to a particular HLA-DQ α/β heterodimer. *J. Exp. Med.* **169**: 345–350.

Spielman, R.S., Baker, L. and Zmijewski, C.M. (1979). Inheritance of susceptibility to juvenile onset diabetes. *Prog. Clin. Biol. Res.* **32**: 567–585.

Spies, T., Blanck, G., Bresnahan, M. et al. (1989). A new cluster of genes within the human major histocompatibility complex. *Science* **243**: 214–217.

Srikanta, S., Ganda, O.P., Eisenbarth, G.S. et al. (1983). Islet cell antibodies and beta cell function in monozygotic triplets and twins initially discordant for Type I diabetes mellitus. *N. Engl. J. Med.* **308**: 322–325.

Suarez, B., Hodge, S.E. and Reich, T. (1979). Is juvenile diabetes determined by a single gene closely linked to HLA? *Diabetes* **28**: 527–532.

Svejgaard, A., Platz, P. and Ryder, L.P. (1983). HLA and Disease 1982 – a survey. *Immunol. Rev.* **70**: 193–218.

Szafer, F., Brautbar, C., Tzfoni, E. et al. (1987). Detection of disease-specific restriction fragment length polymorphisms in pemphigus vulgaris linked to the DQw1 and DQw3 alleles of the HLA-D region. *Prot. Natl Acad. Sci. USA* **84**: 6542–6545.

Tanaka, S., Nakajima, S., Inoue, S. et al. (1990). Genetic control by I-A subregion in H-2 comlex of incidence of streptozotocin-induced autoimmune diabetes in mice. *Diabetes* **39**: 1298–1304.

Taurog, J.D. and El-Zaatari, F.A.K. (1988). In vitro mutagenesis of HLA-B27. Substitution of an unpaired cysteine residue in the α1 domain causes loss of antibody-defined epitopes. *J. Clin. Invest.* **82**: 987–992.

Theofilopoulos, A.N. and Dixon, F.J. (1981). Etiopathogenesis of murine SLE. *Immun. Rev.* **55**: 179–216.

Thomsen, M., Platz, P., Christy, M. et al. (1979). HLA-D-associated resistance and susceptibility to insulin-dependent diabetes mellitus. *Transplant. Proc.* **11**: 1307–1308.

Thomson, G. (1980). A two-locus model for juvenile diabetes. *Ann. Hum. Genet.* **43**: 383–398.

Thorsby, E., Helgesen, A., Solheim, B.G. et al. (1977). HLA antigens in multiple sclerosis. *J. Neurol. Sci.* **32**: 187–193.

Tiwari, J.L., Betuel, H., Gebuhrer, L. et al. (1984). Genetic epidemiology of coeliac disease. *Genet. Epidemiol.* **1**: 37–42.

Tiwari, J.L. and Terasaki, P.I. (1985). *HLA and Disease Associations*. Springer Verlag, New York.

Todd, J.A., Acha-Orbea, H., Bell, J.I. et al. (1988a). A molecular basis for MHC Class II-associated autoimmunity. *Science* **240**: 1003–1009.

Todd, J.A., Bell, J.I. and McDevitt, H.O. (1988b). A molecular basis for genetic susceptibility to insulin-dependent diabetes mellitus. *Trends Genet.* **4**: 129–134.

Todd, J.A., Fukui, Y., Kitagawa, T. et al. (1990). The A3 allele of the HLA-DQA1 locus is associated with susceptibility to type I diabetes in Japanese. *Proc. Natl Acad. Sci. USA* **87**: 1094–1098.

Traugott, U., Reinherz, E.L. and Raine, C.S. (1983). Multiple sclerosis: distribution of T cell subsets within active chronic lesions. *Science* **219**: 308–310.

Tsuchiya, N., Husby, G. and Williams, R.C. (1989). Studies of humoral and cell-mediated immunity to peptides shared by HLA-B27.1 and *Klebsiella pneumoniae* nitrogenase in ankylosing spondylitis. *Clin. Exp. Immunol.* **76**: 354–360.

Urban, J.L., Kumar, V., Kono, D.H. et al. (1988). Restricted use of T cell receptor V genes in murine autoimmune encephalomyelitis raises possibilities for antibody therapy. *Cell* **54**: 577–592.

Vague, P. (1984). *Frontiers in Diabetes*, Vol 4, *Diabetes mellitus: Etiopathogenesis and Metabolic Aspects* (eds F. Belfiore, D.J. Galton and G.M. Reaven), pp. 12–25, Karger, Basel.

van den Berg-Loonen, E.M., Nijenhuis, L.E., Engelfriet, C.P. et al. (1977). Segregation of HLA haplotypes in 100 families with a myasthenia gravis patient. *J. Immunogenet.* **4**: 331–340.

Vartdal, F., Sollid, L.M., Vandvik, B. et al. (1989). Patients with multiple sclerosis carry DQB1 genes which encode shared polymorphic aminoacid-sequences. *Hum. Immunol.* **25**: 103–110.

Walford, R.L., Finkelstein, S., Neerhout, R. et al. (1970). Acute childhood leukaemia in relation to the HL-A human transplantation genes. *Nature* **225**: 461–463.

Watanabe, Y., Tokunaga, K., Matsuki, K. et al. (1989). Putative amino acid sequence of HLA-DRB chain contributing to rheumatoid arthritis susceptibility. *J. Exp. Med.* **169**: 2263–2268.

Wolf, E., Spencer, K.M. and Cudworth, A.G. (1983). The genetic susceptibility to type I (insulin-dependent) diabetes. Analysis of the HLA-DR association. *Diabetologia* **24**: 224–230.

Wong, S., Moore, S., Orisio, S. et al. (1991). Susceptibility to type 1 diabetes in women is associated with the CD3 epsilon locus on chromosome 11. *Clin. Exp. Immunol.* **83**: 69–73.

Woodroofe, M.N., Bellamy, A.S., Feldmann, M. et al. (1986). Immunocytochemical characterisation of the immune reaction in the central nervous system in multiple sclerosis. *J. Neurol. Sci.* **74**: 135–152.

Wordsworth, B.P., Lanchbury, J.S. and Sakkas, L.I. (1989). HLA-DR4 subtype frequencies in rheumatoid arthritis indicate that DRB1 is the major susceptibility locus within the HLA class II region. *Proc. Natl Acad. Sci. USA* **86**: 10049–10053.

Wraith, D.C., McDevitt, H.O., Steinman, L. et al. (1989). T cell recognition as the target for immune intervention in autoimmune disease. *Cell* **57**: 709–715.

Yamagata, K., Nakajima, H., Hanafusa, T. et al. (1989). Aspartic acid at position 57 of DQβ chain does not protect against type I (insulin-dependent) diabetes mellitus in Japanese subjects. *Diabetologia* **32**: 762–764.

Yoon, J.W., Austin, M., Onodera, T. et al. (1979). Virus-induced diabetes mellitus. Isolation of a virus from the pancreas of a child with diabetic ketoacidosis. *N. Engl. J. Med.* **300**: 1173–1179.

Zamvil, S.S., Mitchell, D.J., Lee, N.E. et al. (1988). Predominant expression of a T cell receptor Vβ gene subfamily in autoimmune encephalomyelitis. *J. Exp. Med.* **167**: 1586–1596

Zvaifler, N.J. (1988). New perspectives on the pathogenesis of rheumatoid arthritis. *Am. J. Med.* **85**: 12–17.

CHAPTER 8
Connective tissue diseases

Mark Walport
Department of Rheumatology
Royal Postgraduate Medical School
London, UK

Introduction

Three groups of genes encoded within the MHC are attractive candidates as disease susceptibility genes for connective tissue diseases, some of which are thought to be mediated by immune complexes, such as SLE. These are the HLA class II genes, complement genes of the class III region and other genes within the class III region, such as those encoding tumour necrosis factor. Initial studies established that there was a raised prevalence of the HLA products HLA-B8, -DR3 and -DR2 amongst cohorts of Caucasian patients with systemic lupus erythematosus (SLE), compared to controls. Subsequent studies showed that a particular haplotype, HLA-A1,-B8, -DR3, is particularly common amongst Caucasian patients with SLE. Dissection of the relevant gene within this haplotype has proved a difficult problem and, although a deleted allele for C4A (i.e. partial inherited C4A deficiency) is presently the strongest candidate as a disease susceptibility gene, uncertainty still remains.

The theme of this chapter is an analysis of the approaches that have been taken to identify particular disease susceptibility genes within the HLA region whose products (or lack of them) may increase the chances of the development of SLE and related diseases. The arguments used may be generally applied to the analysis of the associations of polymorphisms of particular loci with disease. The other diseases to be considered in this chapter are 1° Sjögren's syndrome, polymyositis and systemic sclerosis, each of which is associated with the production of autoantibodies to intracellular antigens. The common denominator of these autoantigens is functional – the majority take part in the transcription of nucleic acids and their translation into protein. There is strong evidence that the autoantibodies of SLE play a role in disease causation mediated by the formation of immune complexes with the relevant autoantigen. In contrast, in polymyositis and systemic sclerosis, it is more likely that

HLA and Disease
ISBN 0–12–440320–4

the autoantibodies are bystanders which provide an unsolved clue to aetiology though not to pathogenesis.

Complement proteins of the Class III region

C4, encoded by the two tandemly duplicated genes, C4A and C4B, shows the highest degree of polymorphism of all the complement proteins. Tandem duplication may increase the probability of generation of polymorphism by such mechanisms as gene conversion and extensive polymorphism is seen in other tandemly duplicated genes.

The structural variants of C4A and of C4B can be detected by differences in electrophoretic mobility (Awdeh and Alper, 1980). Included in the polymorphisms of C4A and C4B are null variants (usually expressed as C4AQ*0 or C4BQ*0, i.e. quantity zero) for which no protein product may be detected. Up to 30% of normal Caucasoid subjects may have a single C4 null allele. Approximately 4% of Caucasoid populations show homozygous C4A deficiency and 1% have homozygous C4B deficiency. Alloantibodies to C4A and C4B may arise amongst such individuals following transfusion, which may be detected as haemagglutinins (normal erythrocytes bear small numbers of covalently fixed C4d molecules). Alloantibodies to C4A and C4B occasionally arise in subjects with C4A or C4B deficiencies who have received transfusions. These were originally characterized as the blood groups Rodgers and Chido and later correlated with antigens located on C4A and C4B, respectively (O'Neill et al., 1978).

The molecular basis for the commonest C4 null allele, C4AQ*0, inherited in the common Caucasoid MHC haplotype HLA-A1, B8, DR3, C4AQ*0, C4B1, C2–1, BfS, has been shown to be due to a deletion of the C4A gene (Carroll et al., 1985; Yu and Campbell, 1987). Other haplotypes include three C4 genes and this suggests that mismatched crossovers may be responsible for the variation in C4 gene number in humans. A further C4A polymorphic variant, C4A6, is unusual in that it is haemolytically inactive. This variant has been purified and shown to be active in the formation of a C3- but not a C5-convertase enzyme (Dodds et al., 1985; Kinoshita et al., 1989). The structural basis of this abnormality has recently been shown to be due to an Arg to Trp substitution at position 458 in the β chain of C4A6 (Anderson et al., 1992).

C2 and Factor B, probable gene duplicates and close functional relatives, are also encoded in the MHC closely linked to C4A and C4B (Carroll et al., 1984). Both of these proteins show common inherited polymorphisms, which in the case of C2 also includes a null allele. This null allele is almost invariably encoded in a Caucasian haplotype with a prevalence of 1% to 2%, HLA-A10(A25), B18, DR2, C4A*4, C4B*2, C2*Q0, BfS (Hauptmann et al., 1982). Homozygous C2 deficiency is by far the commonest homozygous complement deficiency encountered in Caucasian populations and has a prevalence of approximately 1:10 000 (reviewed in Ruddy, 1986).

The two isotypes of C4 show subtle functional differences; C4A binding better to immune complexes and C4B being haemolytically more active. These functional differences are explained by a difference in the susceptibility to nucleophilic attack by the two isotypes. C4A preferentially binds to amine groups, abundantly present in proteins, whereas C4B binds preferentially to hydroxyl groups which are pre-dominantly found in carbohydrates (Isenman and Young, 1984; Law et al., 1984). More carbohydrate than amine groups are available for the binding of C4 on erythrocytes, which explains the greater haemolytic activity of C4B than C4A. The major consistent differences between the proteins encoded by the C4A and C4B genes lie at amino-acid positions, 1101, 1102, 1105 and 1106 [C4A Pro, Cys, Leu and Asp; C4B Leu, Ser, Ile and His (Yu et al., 1986)]. Carroll and co-workers (1990) showed, using site-directed mutagenesis, that conversion of Asp 1106 to His changed the reactivity of a genetically-engineered C4B to that of C4A with respect to binding properties.

Complement deficiency and immune-complex disease

Homozygous complement deficiency and SLE

A gene may be associated with expression of disease either because its product is directly relevant to disease causation or because it is closely linked to the relevant gene. The observation that the same disease association is found with products of two or more genes which share similar physiological activities but are encoded on different chromosomes strongly implies a causative link between those gene products and disease susceptibility. This is well illustrated by the association of inherited deficiencies of the complement system and SLE. Hereditary homozygous deficiencies of C1q and C4 are each associated with a greater than 75% prevalence of SLE and homozygous deficiency of C2 with an approximately 33% prevalence of SLE (Lachmann and Walport, 1987). Such patients only account for a tiny minority of all patients with SLE but may give a very important clue to one of the pathogenetic factors. Complement components C4 and C2 are encoded within the MHC and C1q is encoded by three genes located on a 24 kb stretch of DNA on chromosome 1p (Sellar et al., 1991). Although C4 is encoded within the MHC, null alleles of both C4A and C4B appear to have arisen sporadically in several different MHC haplotypes (Hauptmann et al., 1986) and because of this it seems unlikely that linked MHC genes are responsible for disease susceptibility in the context of homozygous C4 deficiency. This argument cannot be applied so easily to C2 deficiency, which is usually inherited in a particular haplotype, HLA-A10, -B18, -DR2, C2Q*0 (Fu and Kunkel, 1975).

C4 null alleles and SLE

Having established a link between homozygous complement deficiency and SLE, the hypothesis was formulated that partial inherited complement deficiency might also cause increased disease susceptibility. It was discovered that C4A and C4B, the two isotypes of C4 encoded in tandem within the MHC, were both highly polymorphic and that the polymorphism included null alleles (designated Q*0) at both loci. This led to a test of the hypothesis that the disease susceptibility locus within the MHC might be null alleles of one or both loci of C4 (studies reviewed in Tables 8.1 and 8.2).

Initial studies showed that there was indeed an increased prevalence of null alleles,

Table 8.1   Prevalence of homozygous deficiency of C4A or C4B amongst different populations of patients with SLE

Reference	Ethnic group	Homozygous C4A deficiency				Homozygous C4B deficiency			
		Patients		Controls		Patients		Controls	
		%	n[a]	%	n	%	n	%	n
1	Caucasoid	14	29	0	42	0	29	0	42
2	Caucasoid	12	41	0	176	5	41	4	176
3	Caucasoid	10	88	2	236	–	–	–	–
4	Caucasoid	13	15	0	63	7	15	3	63
5	Caucasoid	11	63	0	63	–	–	–	–
6	Caucasoid	8	63	1.5	197	3	63	4	197
7	Caucasoid	7	27[b]	5	144[b]	0	27	1	144
6	Chinese	2	75	0	76	0	75	0	76
6	Japanese	12	61	0	50	0	51	0	51
5	Black	1	35	0	35	–	–	–	–

[a] Total number of subjects tested.   [b] no of haplotypes studied.
Reference: 1 = Fielder et al. (1983); 2 = Christiansen et al. (1983); 3 = Kemp et al. (1987); 4 = Reveille et al. (1985); 5 = Howard et al. (1986); 6 = Dunckley et al. (1987); 7 = Schur et al (1990)

mainly of C4A, amongst Caucasian patients with SLE but the analysis was confounded by strong linkage disequilibrium between C4A null alleles and HLA-DR3 (Fielder et al., 1983). This effectively prevented separation of the relative contribution of these two putative disease susceptibility genes.

Is the relevant gene C4A Q*0 or HLA-DR3?

Two approaches have been used to attempt to disentangle the relative contributions of HLA-DR3 and C4A Q*0 to disease susceptibility. The first is examination of the HLA associations with SLE in different racial groups in which haplotypes containing different combinations of the allotypic variants of the different HLA gene products are found. Using this type of approach, it has been found that the association of SLE with HLA-DR3 breaks down, but the association with C4A Q*0 is sustained (Tables 8.1 and 8.2) with the exception of a study by Schur and colleagues (1990). This finding is most striking in Japanese populations amongst whom HLA-DR3 is extremely rare. The second approach is to select patients who are DR3-negative to test the hypothesis that in this subgroup of individuals the prevalence of C4A Q*0 alleles remains elevated. The results of such a study were more ambiguous – there was a statistically significant elevation of the prevalence of C4A Q*0 and C4B Q*0 alleles together but not of C4 AQ*0 alleles alone (Batchelor et al., 1987).

Physiological arguments for the link between complement deficiency and SLE

The explanation for the link between complement deficiency and increased susceptibility to SLE is not certain. It has been known since work by Heidelberger in the 1940s that complement activation by immune complexes interferes with lattice formation and tends to maintain immune complexes in solution (Heidelberger, 1941). When

Table 8.2   Prevalence of HLA-DR2 and -DR3 amongst different populations of patients with SLE

Reference	Ethnic group	HLA-DR2 frequency				HLA-DR3 frequency			
		Patients		Controls		Patients		Controls	
		% positive	n[a]	% positive	n	% positive	n	% positive	n
1	Caucasoid[b]	**57**	28	26	490	**46**	28	22	490
2	Caucasoid[b]	**50**	24	25	40	**54**	24	20	40
3	Caucasoid[b]	20	40	28	123	**43**	40	11	123
4	Caucasoid[b]	**53**	30	26	258	37	30	17	258
5	Caucasoid[b]	21	28	20	125	39	28	16	125
6	Caucasoid[b]	**38**	106	23	132	37	106	30	132
7	Caucasoid[b]	**44**	111	24	626	33	111	25	626
8	Caucasoid[c]	20	46	28	134	**54**	46	36	134
9	Caucasoid[b]	**46**	63	22	63	38	63	25	63
10	Caucasoid[b]	**41**	217	29	1926	**41**	217	23	1926
11	Caucasoid[c]	21	49	11	56	**30**	49	13	56
12	Japanese[b]	**51**	45	25	36	0	45	0	36
13	Japanese[b]	**47**	86	21	75	0	86	1.3	75
14	Japanese[c]	**50**	38	21	75				
15	N.Chinese[b]	**69**	26	33	405				
16	S.Chinese[b]	**62**	100	38	100	9	100	8	100
4	Black[b]	48	25	30	73	48	25	32	73
5	Black[b]	25	36	33	168	28	36	25	168
6	Black[b]	26	35	26	35	31	35	26	35
17	Black[b]	32	31	38	73	**58**	31	27	73
18	Black[b]	**41**	37	18	147	**62**	37	20	117
19	Black[b]	29	28	23	137	36	28	25	137
20	Black[c]	46	63	40	57	33	63	34	57

[a] Total number of subjects tested.
[b] DR type ascertained by serological typing.
[c] DR type ascertained by DNA typing.
Bold figures denote significant associations (Chi-square analysis, not corrected for number of comparisons)
References: 1 = Reinertsen et al. (1978); 2 = Gibofsky et al. (1978); 3 = Celada et al. (1980); 4 = Gladman et al. (1979); 5 = Scherak et al. (1980); 6 = Schur et al. (1982); 7 = Hochberg et al. (1985); 8 = Dunckley et al. (1986); 9 = Howard et al. (1986); 10 = Hartung et al. (1989); 11 So et al. (1990); 12 = Kameda et al. (1982); 13 = Hashimoto et al. (1985); 14 = Dunckley et al. (1985); 15 = Naito et al. (1986); 16 = Hawkins et al. (1987); 17 = Alarif et al. (1983); 18 = Kachru et al. (1984); 19 = Wilson et al. (1984); 20 = Reveille et al. (1989)

immune complexes are formed in the presence of complement, precipitation is inhibited. This is particularly a property of the classical pathway of complement. In contrast, the alternative pathway of complement is implicated in solubilizing pre-formed immune complexes (Schifferli et al., 1982). The prevalence and severity of SLE associated with inherited complement deficiency is highest for C1q followed by C4 and then C2. This implies a physiological link between disease induction and an activity of the classical pathway of complement. Inhibition of immune precipitation may be the relevant activity and it has been proposed that complement deficiency leads to ineffective processing of immune complexes, followed by defective clearance of complexes by the mononuclear phagocytic system (Lachmann and Walport, 1987). This allows deposition of immune complexes in tissues causing inflammation. This inflammation leads in turn to release of autoantigens and the stimulation of a self-perpetuating autoantibody response. Some evidence in support of this hypothesis has come from studies of the mechanisms of immune complex clearance in rabbits, monkeys and man (Haakenstad and Mannik, 1974; Waxman et al., 1984; Schifferli et al., 1989).

A second hypothesis to link complement deficiency with SLE flows from a role of the complement system in host defence against infectious disease. There is unequivocal evidence that deficiency of classical pathway proteins is linked with increased susceptibility to infections by pyogenic bacteria, but no evidence for a role for such bacteria in causation of SLE. In contrast there is little clear evidence linking complement deficiency to increased susceptibility to virus infections. However, complement is effective in lysis of certain retrovirally infected cells (though not HIV-infected cells). There is enthusiasm for a possible role for retroviruses in the induction of SLE, though little hard evidence. It may be postulated that complement deficiency could promote infection by some, as yet unrecognized, viral agent.

Are null alleles of C4A the only disease susceptibility gene for SLE in the MHC?

The role of HLA-DR2 and -DR3

Many studies have been performed examining the prevalence of different MHC class I and II allotypic variants in patients with SLE (summarized in Walport et al., 1982; Hartung et al., 1989) (Table 8.2). From these many studies it appears that the two dominant associations amongst Caucasian patients, especially Europeans, are with the haplotype HLA-A1, -B8, -DR3, -DQw2 and with HLA-DR2, -DQw1. The excess of HLA-DR3 may be almost entirely due to its linkage with C4A Q*0 alleles. However, the same is not the case for HLA-DR2 which is often not associated with a null allele of C4A, and appears to function in some populations as an independent risk factor (Howard et al., 1986). This suggests that either HLA-DR2, or a polymorphic product encoded by a gene in strong linkage disequilibrium with DR2, may also function as a disease susceptibility gene. The complexity of the problem is shown in Table 8.2 where it may be seen that, amongst Caucasian populations, HLA-DR2 and -DR3 are found in excess; amongst Chinese and Japanese populations, only HLA-DR2 alone is found with an increased frequency; and in black populations, no significant excess of any HLA-DR product has been detected in the majority of studies.

TNF genes and SLE

There are intriguing data suggesting possible links between the TNF-α gene and SLE. (NZB × NZW) F_1 mice suffer from severe nephritis, not seen in the parental NZB strain, in which the dominant disease manifestation is autoimmune haemolytic anaemia. NZW mice were found to produce low levels of TNF-α and treatment of the (NZB × NZW) F_1 hybrid strain with TNF-α was associated with delay in onset of nephritis and prolonged survival (Jacob and McDevitt, 1988). Supporting evidence of genetic variation in, or near, the TNF-α gene was provided by the finding of an RFLP using a TNF-α cDNA probe, found in NZW, BXSB, MRL/lpr and some non-autoimmune strains of mice. The relevance of this RFLP to the reduced TNF-α production in NZW mice is doubtful, as BXSB and MRL/lpr mice, which share the same RFLP, do not show reduced TNF-α production (Jacob et al., 1990). Polymorphisms around the TNF-α genes have also been described in humans, and variation in mitogen-stimulated TNF-α production (but not TNF-β) was correlated with HLA-DR type (Jacob et al., 1990). Subjects with HLA-DR3 or -DR4 were found to be high producers of TNF-α whereas HLA-DR2-positive individuals were low producers. A correlation has been reported between the prevalence of lupus nephritis and the presence of HLA-DR2 (Fronek et al., 1988), though further data are needed to substantiate this association. If this were the case, it would raise the possibility that the clinical manifestations of SLE may be influenced by the presence of abnormally high (DR3) or low (DR2) levels of TNF-α.

Do Ir genes exist for autoantibody production?

It has been postulated that there is genetic control of the expression of particular autoantibodies. Clear evidence for such control comes from breeding experiments conducted in murine strains susceptible to SLE-like disease, and non-MHC-linked genes are probably involved. The situation in human disease is not clear in that there are differences in prevalence of particular autoantibodies in patients of different races. For example, the prevalence of anti-Sm antibodies is about 25% in black (Arnett et al., 1988), Chinese (Boey et al., 1988) and Japanese (Yokohari and Tsunematsu, 1985) patients compared with approximately 10% in Caucasian patients with SLE (Arnett et al., 1988; Bernstein et al., 1984).

There is evidence that different class II MHC genes are associated with a raised prevalence of particular autoantibodies, for example, HLA-DR3 with anti-Ro and anti-La antibodies (Bell and Maddison, 1980; Manthorpe et al., 1982), and HLA-DR4 with anti-RNP antibodies (Genth et al., 1987). There is related evidence that the level of anti-Ro and anti-La antibodies may be higher in individuals who are heterozygous for HLA-DQw1/-DQw2 (Harley et al., 1986; Hamilton et al., 1988) raising the possibility that hybrid DQ molecules (DQw1α/DQw2β or DQw1β/DQw2α) may be relevant. It has been proposed that the class II genes may function directly as immune response (Ir) genes. However, anti-Ro and anti-La antibodies are a common feature of SLE that is associated with homozygous deficiency of C4, which as has been discussed above, shows no constant association with any particular MHC class II molecules (Meyer et al., 1985).

A related question is whether HLA-encoded genes influence the pattern of disease. Conflicting data have been reported (reviewed in Table 8.3). There is good agreement that the A1,B8,DR3 haplotype is particularly associated with subacute cutaneous lupus erythematosus, neonatal lupus and 1° Sjögren's syndrome, and each of these in turn is associated with the presence of anti-Ro and anti-La antibodies. Similarly, there is an increasing body of evidence supporting an association between DR4 and mixed connective tissue disease (MCTD) with anti-RNP antibodies (Genth et al., 1987). There is conflicting evidence about possible associations of renal lupus with any particular HLA product or haplotype. A positive association with DR2 (Fronek et al., 1988), a positive association with A1,B8 (Rigby et al., 1978), or no MHC association (Ahearn et al., 1982) have all been reported.

Table 8.3   The published associations of different MHC products with particular subsets of disease or autoantibodies

Antibody or disease association	MHC association	Reference
subacute cutaneous LE	DR3	Sontheimer et al. (1982)
1° Sjögren's syndrome	DR3	Chused et al. (1977)
anti-Ro	DR3	Bell and Maddison (1980)
anti-Ro, anti-La	DR3	Hochberg et al. (1985)
anti-Ro, anti-La	DR2,DQ1/DR3,DQ2 heterozygous (SLE)	Hamilton et al. (1988)
anti-Ro, anti-La	DR2,DQ1/DR3,DQ2 heterozygous (1° SS)	Harley et al. (1986)
anti-nDNA, anti-ssDNA antibodies	DR2	Alvarellos et al. (1983)
renal disease, anti-nDNA antibodies	DR2	Fronek et al. (1990)
severe disease with nephritis	A1,B8 (linkage disequ with DR3)	Rigby et al. (1978)
mild disease, little nephritis	A2,B7 (linkage disequ with DR2)	Rigby et al. (1978)
anti-nDNA	DR3	Griffing et al. (1980)
anti-nDNA, anti-Sm	DR7	Schur et al. (1982)
anti-nDNA	nil (whites), DR2 (blacks)	Hochberg et al. (1985)
anti-nDNA	nil	Smolen et al. (1987)
anti-nRNP, -Sn	DR4	Smolen et al. (1987)
anti-nRNP, -Sm	DR2 (weakly associated)	Hamilton et al. (1988)
anti-nRNP, -Sm	DR4	Harley et al. (1989)

Drug-induced lupus

Many drugs have been associated with the development of a disease resembling idiopathic SLE (reviewed in Lee and Chase, 1975), but with a rather different pattern of organ involvement and spectrum of autoantibodies. The presence of anti-histone autoantibodies is typical (Rubin and Waga, 1987). A characteristic of drug-induced lupus is of gradual resolution after withdrawal of the drug. The two commonest causes of this disease are hydralazine, an anti-hypertensive agent, and procainamide, an anti-arrhythmic agent. Lupus associated with both of these two compounds shares certain immunogenetic features, in particular with a genetic polymorphism of the acetyl transferase enzyme associated with slow acetylation of the two drugs. The prevalence of slow drug acetylators is very greatly increased in patients with lupus induced by these drugs in comparison with controls. This observation suggests that the native, rather than the acetylated metabolite of the drug, is associated with pathogenesis. This has been confirmed by the finding that administration of acetyl-procainamide does not cause a flare of lupus in subjects who have previously suffered disease in response to the native drug (Kluger et al., 1981).

It is of note that the HLA associations of drug-induced lupus are different from those of primary SLE; DR4 occurred at an increased prevalence in two groups of patients with hydralazine-induced disease (Batchelor et al., 1980; Mitchell et al., 1987), although this observation was not confirmed in a study of Australian patients (Brand et al., 1984). Sim proposed an hypothesis that hydralazine and procainamide might be linked with the development of SLE by inactivation of C4, due to nucleophilic attack on the internal thioester bond of C4 (Sim et al., 1984). Evidence supporting this hypothesis was collected by Speirs et al. (1989) who studied 21 patients with hydralazine lupus, and found that 16 (76%) had one or more C4 null alleles, compared with a frequency of 43% in a panel of 82 normal subjects. They concluded that, as in idiopathic SLE, hydralazine-induced lupus may depend partly upon genetically determined C4 levels.

1° Sjögren's syndrome

There is a high degree of clinical, serological and immunogenetic overlap between 1° Sjögren's syndrome and SLE, and many of the salient points about the genetics of 1° Sjögren's syndrome have already been considered earlier in the chapter and have recently been reviewed (Davies and Walport, 1990). The strongest association in Caucasian subjects is with HLA-B8,-DR3,-DRw52, though in contrast a study in Japanese patients showed a high prevalence of HLA-DRw53 (Moriuchi et al., 1986), which is the second expressed DR molecule on haplotypes that encode DR4, 7 and 9. Antibodies to Ro and La are one of the dominant serological features of 1° Sjögren's syndrome, and the studies of Harley and his collaborators relating high expression of these antibodies to heterozygosity for HLA-DQw1/-DQw2 have been reviewed above. A possible role for class III products in disease susceptibility to 1° Sjögren's syndrome has not been established.

Polymyositis and dermatomyositis

Both the juvenile and adult inflammatory myopathies have been associated in Caucasian populations with the HLA-A1,-B8,-DR3,-C4AQ*0 haplotype (Behan et al., 1978; Hirsch et al., 1981; Friedman et al., 1983; Robb et al., 1988). This association appeared to be particularly strong in the subset of polymyositis patients with interstitial pulmonary fibrosis and autoantibodies to aminoacyl tRNA synthetase enzymes (Jo-1, PL-7 and PL-12) (Hirsch et al., 1981; Goldstein et al., 1990). No association with DR3 was found in two studies of adult black patients with polymyositis (Goldstein et al., 1990; Moulds et al., 1990). The only class II gene product which was present at raised prevalence in both racial groups was DRw52, a serological specificity related to the DRB3 gene, and found on haplotypes bearing DR3,-5,-w6 and -w8 (Goldstein et al., 1990). These DRB1 genes associated with DRw52 share a polymorphic sequence located in the first hypervariable region and this constitutes part of the 'floor' of the class II molecule, in the peptide binding groove (deduced by analogy with the known crystallographic structure of HLA-class I). Possible mechanisms by which such sequences contribute to disease susceptibility are considered in Chapters 3–5. There is some evidence against a role for class III gene in disease susceptibility to polymyositis, in that there was only a slight increase (not statistically significant) in the prevalence of C4AQ*0 alleles in 35 black patients; 31% had C4AQ*0 compared with 20% controls (Moulds et al., 1990).

Systemic sclerosis

No consistent picture has emerged of any particular HLA association with systemic sclerosis and its variants, and the conflicting data have recently been reviewed by

Briggs and colleagues (1990). HLA-DR1,-DR3 and -DR5 have mainly been implicated in studies of white patients and DR2 and DR4 in Japanese subjects. Attempts
to clarify the analysis by classification of patients according to type of disease,
systemic or limited (CREST), or by antibody, anti-centromere or anti-topoisomerase 1
(Genth et al., 1990), have not produced consistent results. Similarly, although an
association with C4 null alleles has been reported in Caucasian populations by one
group (Briggs et al., 1990), this was not confirmed by another (Livingston et al.,
1987).

Conclusions

The extreme polymorphism of the genes of the MHC, the large number of different
genes expressing products with diverse function, coupled with linkage disequilibrium,
conspire to hinder the precise identification of the disease susceptibility genes which
undoubtedly exist within this portion of the genome. The most intense endeavour has
been directed to analysis of the structure, function and associations of MHC class I
and II alleles with disease susceptibility. The analysis of the HLA associations with
SLE and related diseases has suggested the possibility of other genes within this region
(most importantly complement and TNF genes) also playing a role in increasing
susceptibility to diseases mediated by disturbances of the immune system.

References

Ahearn, J.M., Provost, T.T., Dorsch, C.A. et al. (1982). Interrelationships of HLA-DR, MB and MT
 phenotypes, autoantibody expression, and clinical features in systemic lupus erythrematosus. *Arthritis
 Rheum.* **25**: 1031–1040.
Alarif, L.I., Ruppert, G.B., Wilson, R., Jr. et al. (1983). HLA-DR antigens in Blacks with rheumatoid
 arthritis and systemic lupus erythematosus. *J. Rheumatol.* **10**: 297–300.
Alvarellos, A., Ahearn, J.M., Provost, T.T. et al. (1983). Relationships of HLA-DR and MT antigens to
 autoantibody expression in systemic lupus erythematosus. *Arthritis Rheum.* **26**: 1533–1535 (letter).
Anderson, M.J., Milner, C.M., Cotton, R.G.H. et al. (1992). The coding sequence of the hemolytically
 inactive C4A6 allotype of human complement component C4 reveals that a single arginine to tryptophan
 substitution at b-chain residue 458 is the likely cause of the defect. *J. Immunol.* **148**: 2795–2802.
Arnett, F.C., Hamilton, R.G., Roebber, M.G. et al. (1988). Increased frequencies of Sm and nRNP
 autoantibodies in American blacks compared to whites with systemic lupus erythematosus. *J. Rheumatol.*
 15: 1773–1776.
Awdeh, Z.L. and Alper, C.A. (1980). Inherited structural polymorphism of the fourth component of
 human complement. *Proc. Natl Acad. Sci. USA* **77**: 3576–3580.
Batchelor, J.R., Welsh, K.I. and Tinoco, R.M. (1980). Hydralazine-induced systemic lupus erythematosus:
 influence of HLA-DR and sex on susceptibility. *Lancet* **1**: 1107–1109.
Batchelor, J.R., Fielder, A.H., Walport, M.J. et al. (1987). Family study of the major histocompatibility
 complex in HLA DR3 negative patients with systemic lupus erythematosus. *Clin. Exp. Immunol.* **70**:
 364–371.
Behan, W.M., Behan, P.O. and Dick, H.A. (1978). HLA-B8 in polymyositis. *N. Engl. J. Med.* **298**: 1260–1261.
Bell, D.A. and Maddison, P.J. (1980). Serologic subsets in systemic lupus erythematosus. *Arthritis Rheum.*
 23: 1268–1273.
Bernstein, R.M., Bunn, C.C., Hughes, G.R.V. et al. (1984). Cellular protein and RNA antigens in
 autoimmune disease. *Mol. Biol. Med.* **2**: 105–120.

Boey, M.L., Peebles, C.L., Tsay, G. et al. (1988). Clinical and autoantibody correlations in Orientals with systemic lupus erythematosus. *Ann. Rheum. Dis.* **47**: 918–923.

Brand, C., Davidson, A., Littlejohn, G. et al. (1984). Hydralazine-induced lupus: no association with HLA-DR4. *Lancet* **1**: 462.

Briggs, D., Black, C. and Welsh, K. (1990). Genetic factors in scleroderma. *Rheum. Dis. Clin. North Am.* **16**: 31–50.

Carroll, M.C., Campbell, R.D., Bentley, D.R. et al. (1984). A molecular map of the major histocompatibility complex class III region of man linking complement genes C4, C2 and factor B. *Nature* **307**: 237–241.

Carroll, M.C., Palsdottir, A., Belt, K.T. et al. (1985). Deletion of complement C4 and steroid 21-hydroxylase genes in HLA Class III region. *EMBO J.* **4**: 2547–2552.

Carroll, M.C., Fathallah, D.M., Bergamaschini, L. et al. (1990). Substitution of a single amino acid (aspartic acid for histidine) converts the functional activity of human complement C4B to C4A. *Proc. Natl Acad. Sci. USA* **87**: 6868–6872.

Celada, A., Barras, C., Benzonana, G. et al. (1980). Increased frequency of HLA-DRw3 in systemic lupus erythematosus. *Tissue Antigens* **15**: 283–288

Christiansen, F.T., Dawkins, R.L., Uko, G. et al. (1983). Complement allotyping in SLE: association with C4A null. *Aust. N.Z. J. Med.* **13**: 483–488.

Chused, T.M., Kassan, S.S., Opelz, G. et al. (1977). Sjogren's syndrome association with HLA-Dw3. *N. Engl. J. Med.* **296**: 895–897.

Davies, K.A.A. and Walport, M.J. (1990). The immunogenetic basis of Sjögren's syndrome. In *Immunogenetics of Autoimmune Disease* (ed. N.R. Farid), pp. 77–91, CRC Press, Boca Raton, Fl.

Dodds, A.W., Law, S.K. and Porter, R.R. (1985). The origin of the very variable haemolytic activities of the common human complement component C4 allotypes including C4–A6. *EMBO J.* **4**: 2239–2244.

Dunckley, H., Gatenby, P.A. and Serjeantson, S.W. (1986a). DNA typing of HLA-DR antigens in systemic lupus erythematosus. *Immunogenetics* **24**: 158–162.

Dunckley, H., Naito, S. and Serjeantson, S.W. (1986b). DNA-DR typing of Japanese systemic lupus erythematosus patients. In *HLA in Asia-Oceania 1986* (ed. M. Aizawa), pp. 419–422, Hokkaido University Press, Saporo.

Dunckley, H., Gatenby, P.A., Hawkins, B. et al. (1987). Deficiency of C4A is a genetic determinant of systemic lupus erythematosus in three ethnic groups. *J. Immunogenet.* **14**: 209–218.

Fielder, A.H.L., Walport, M.J., Batchelor, J.R. et al. (1983). Family study of the major histocompatibility complex in patients with systemic lupus erythematosus: importance of null alleles of C4A and C4B in determining disease susceptibility. *Br. Med. J.* **286**: 425–428.

Friedman, J.M., Pachman, L.M., Marijowski, M.L. et al. (1983). Immunogenetic studies of juvenile dermatomyositis: HLA-DR antigen frequencies. *Arthritis Rheum.* **26**: 214–216.

Fronek, Z., Timmerman, L.A., Alper, C.A. et al. (1988). Major histocompatibility complex associations with systemic lupus erythematosus. *Am. J. Med.* **85**: 42–44.

Fronek, Z., Timmerman, L.A., Alper, C.A. et al. (1990). Major histocompatibility complex genes and susceptibility to systemic lupus erythematosus. *Arthritis Rheum.* **33**: 1542–1553.

Fu, S.M. and Kunkel, H.G. (1975). Association of C2 deficiency and the HL-A haplotype 10, W18. *Transplantation* **20**: 179–180.

Genth, E., Zarnowski, H., Mieran, R. et al. (1987). HLA-DR4 and Gm (1, 3; 5, 21) are associated with U1-nRNP antibody positive connective tissue disease. *Ann. Rheum. Dis.* **46**: 189.

Genth, E., Mierau, R., Genetzky, P. et al. (1990). Immunogenetic associations of scleroderma-related antinuclear antibodies. *Arthritis Rheum.* **33**: 657–665.

Gibofsky, A., Winchester, R.J., Patarroyo, M. et al. (1978). Disease associations of the Ia-like human alloantigens. Contrasting patterns in rheumatoid arthritis and systemic lupus erythematosus. *J. Exp. Med.* **148**: 1728–1732.

Gladman, D.D., Terasaki, P.I., Park, M.S. et al. (1979). Increased frequency of HLA-DRW2 in SLE. *Lancet* **2**: 902.

Goldstein, R., Duvic, M., Targoff, I.N. et al. (1990). HLA-D region genes associated with autoantibody responses to histidyl-transfer RNA synthetase (Jo-1) and other translation-related factors in myositis. *Arthritis Rheum.* **33**: 1240–1248.

Griffing, W.L., Moore, S.B., Luthra, H.S. et al. (1980). Associations of antibodies to native DNA with HLA-DRw3. A possible major histocompatibility complex-linked human immune response gene. *J. Exp. Med.* **152**: 319–325.

Haakenstad, A.O. and Mannik, M. (1974). Saturation of the reticuloendothelial system with soluble immune complexes. *J. Immunol.* **112**:1939–1948.

Hamilton, R.G., Harley, J.B., Bias, W.B. et al. (1988). Two Ro (SS-A) autoantibody responses in systemic lupus erythematosus. Correlation of HLA-DR/DQ specificities with quantitative expression of Ro (SS-A) autoantibody. *Arthritis Rheum.* **31**: 496–505.

Harley, J.B., Reichlin, M., Arnett, F.C. et al. (1986). Gene interaction at HLA-DQ enhances autoantibody production in primary Sjogren's syndrome. *Science* **232**: 1145–1147.

Harley, J.B., Sestak, A.L., Willis, L.G. et al. (1989). A model for disease heterogeneity in systemic lupus erythematosus. *Arthritis Rheum.* **32**: 826–836.

Hartung, K., Fontana, A., Klar, M. et al. (1989). Association of class I, II and III MHC gene products with systemic lupus erythematosus. Results of a Central European multicenter study. *Rheumatol. Int.* **9**: 13–18.

Hashimoto, H., Tsuda, H., Matsumoto, T. et al. (1985). HLA-antigens associated with systemic lupus erythematosus in Japan. *J. Rheumatol.* **12**: 919–923.

Hauptmann, G., Goetz, J., Uring-Lambert, B. et al. (1986). Component deficiencies. 2. The fourth component. *Prog. All.* **39**: 232–249.

Hauptmann, G., Tongiu, M.M., Goetz, J. et al. (1982). Association of the C2-deficiency gene (C2*Q0) with the C4A*4, C4B*2 genes. *J. Immunogen.* **9**: 127–132.

Hawkins, B.R., Wong, K.L., Wong, R.W.S. et al. (1987). Strong association between the major histocompatibility complex and systemic lupus erythematosus in Southern Chinese. *J. Rheumatol.* **14**: 1128–1131.

Heidelberger, M. (1941). Quantitative chemical studies on complement or alexin. I.A. method. *J. Exp. Med.* **73**: 691–694.

Hirsch, T.J., Enlow, R.W., Bias, W.B. et al. (1981). HLA-D related (DR) antigens in various kinds of myositis. *Hum. Immunol.* **3**: 181–186.

Hochberg, M.C., Boyd, R.E., Ahearn, J.M. et al. (1985). Systemic lupus erythematosus: a review of clinico-laboratory features and immunogenetic markers in 150 patients with emphasis on demographic subsets. *Medicine* **64**: 285–295.

Howard, P.F., Hochberg, M.C., Bias, W.B. et al. (1986). Relationship between C4 null genes, HLA-D region antigens, and genetic susceptibility to systemic lupus erythematosus in Caucasian and black Americans. *Am. J. Med.* **81**: 187–193.

Isenman, D. and Young, J.R. (1984). The molecular basis for the differences in immune hemolysis activity of the Chido and Rodgers isotypes of human complement component C4. *J. Immunol.* **132**: 3019–3027.

Jacob, C.O. and McDevitt, H.O. (1988). Tumour necrosis factor-α in murine autoimmune 'lupus' nephritis. *Nature* **331**: 356–358.

Jacob, C.O., Fronek, Z., Lewis, G.D. et al. (1990). Heritable major histocompatibility complex class II-associated differences in production of tumor factor α: Relevance to genetic predisposition to systemic lupus erythematosus. *Proc. Natl Acad. Sci. USA* **87**: 1233–1237.

Kachru, R.B., Sequeira, W., Mittal, K.K. et al. (1984). A significant increase of HLA-DR3 and DR2 in systemic lupus erythematosus among blacks. *J. Rheumatol.* **11**: 471–474.

Kameda, S., Naito, S., Tanaka, K. et al. (1982). HLA antigens of patients with systemic lupus erythematosus in Japan. *Tissue Antigens* **20**: 221–222.

Kemp, M.E., Atkinson, J.P., Skanes, V.M. et al. (1987). Deletion of C4A genes in patients with systemic lupus erythematosus. *Arthritis Rheum.* **30**: 1015–1022.

Kinoshita, T., Dodds, A.W., Law, S.K.A. et al. (1989). The low C5 convertase activity of the C4A6 allotype of human complement component C4. *Biochem. J.* **261**: 743–748.

Kluger, J., Drayer, D.E., Reidenberg, M.M. et al. (1981). Acetylprocainamide therapy in patients with previous procainamide-induced lupus syndrome. *Ann. Intern. Med.* **95**: 18–23.

Lachmann, P.J. and Walport, M.J. (1987). Deficiency of the effector mechanisms of the immune response and autoimmunity. In *Autoimmunity and Autoimmune Disease, Ciba Foundation Symposium, no. 129.* (ed. J. Whelan), pp. 149–171, Wiley, Chichester.

Law, S.K.A., Dodds, A.W. and Porter, R.R. (1984). A comparison of the properties of two classes, C4A and C4B, of the complement component C4. *EMBO J.* **3**: 1819–1823.

Lee, S.L. and Chase, P.H. (1975). Drug-induced systemic lupus erythematosus: a critical review. *Semin. Arthritis Rheum.* **5**: 83–103.

Livingston, J.Z., Scott, T.E., Wigley, F.M. et al. (1987). Systemic sclerosis (scleroderma): clinical, genetic, and serologic subsets. *J. Rheumatol.* **14**: 512–518.

Manthorpe, R., Teppo, A.M., Bendixen, G. et al. (1982). Antibodies to SS-B in chronic inflammatory connective tissue diseases. Relationship with HLA-Dw2 and HLA-Dw3 antigens in primary Sjögren's syndrome. *Arthritis Rheum.* **25**: 662–667.

Meyer, O., Hauptmann, G., Tappeiner, G. et al. (1985). Genetic deficiency of C4, C2 or C1q and lupus syndromes association with anti-Ro (SS-A) antibodies. *Clin. Exp. Immunol.* **62**: 678–684.

Mitchell, J.A., Batchelor, J.R., Chapel, H. et al. (1987). Erythrocyte complement receptor type 1 (CR1) expression and circulating immune complex (CIC) levels in hydralazine-induced SLE. *Clin. Exp Immunol.* **68**: 446–456.

Moriuchi, J., Ichikawa, Y., Takaya, M. et al. (1986). Association between HLA and Sjögren's syndrome in Japanese patients. *Arthritis Rheum.* **29**: 1518–1521.

Moulds, J.M., Rolih, C., Goldstein, R. et al. (1990). C4 null genes in American whites and blacks with myositis. *J. Rheumatol.* **17**: 331–334.

Naito, S., Kong, F.H., Hawkins, B.R. et al. (1986). Joint report: HLA and disease: SLE. In *HLA in Asia-Oceania 1986* (ed. M. Aizawa), pp. 364–367, Hokkaido University Press, Saporo.

O'Neill, G.J., Yang, S.Y., Tegoli, J. et al. (1978). Chido and Rodgers blood groups are distinct antigenic components of human complement C4. *Nature* **273**: 668–670.

Reinertsen, J.L., Klippel, J.H., Johnson, A.H. et al. (1978). B-lymphocyte alloantigens associated with systemic lupus erythematosus. *N. Engl. J. Med.* **299**: 515–518.

Reveille, J.D., Arnett, F.C., Wilson, R.W. et al. (1985). Null alleles of the fourth component of complement and HLA haplotypes in familial systemic lupus erythematosus. *Immunogenetics* **21**: 299–311.

Reveille, J.D., Schrohenloher, R.E., Acton, R.T. et al. (1989). DNA analysis of HLA-DR and DQ genes in American blacks with systemic lupus erythematosus. *Arthritis Rheum.* **32**: 1243–1251.

Rigby, R.J., Dawkins, R.L., Wetherall, J.D. et al. (1978). HLA in systemic lupus erythematosus: influence on severity. *Tissue Antigens* **12**: 25–31.

Robb, S.A., Fielder, A.H., Saunders, C.E. et al. (1988). C4 complement allotypes in juvenile dermato-myositis. *Hum. Immunol.* **22**: 31–38.

Rubin, R.L. and Waga, S. (1987). Antihistone antibodies in systemic lupus erythematosus. *J. Rheumatol.* **14**: 118–126.

Ruddy, S. (1986). Component deficiencies 3. The second component. *Progr. All.* **39**: 250–266.

Scherak, O., Smolen, J.S. and Mayr, W.R. (1980). HLA-DRw3 and systemic lupus erythematosus. *Arthritis Rheum.* **23**: 954–957.

Schifferli, J.A., Woo, P. and Peters, D.K. (1982). Complement-mediated inhibition of immune precipitation. Role of the classical and alternative pathways. *Clin. Exp. Immunol.* **47**: 555–562.

Schifferli, J.A., Ng, Y.C., Paccaud, J.P. et al. (1989). The role of hypocomplementaemia and low erythrocyte complement receptor type 1 numbers in determining abnormal immune complex clearance in humans. *Clin. Exp. Immunol.* **75**: 329–335.

Schur, P.H., Meyer, I., Garovoy, M. et al. (1982). Associations between systemic lupus erythematosus and the major histocompatibility complex: clinical and immunological considerations. *Clin. Immunol. Immunopathol.* **24**: 263–275.

Schur, P.H., Marcus-Bagley, D., Awdeh, Z. et al. (1990). The effect of ethnicity on major histocompatibility complex complement allotypes and extended haplotypes in patients with systemic lupus erythematosus. *Arthritis Rheum.* **33**: 985–992.

Sellar, G.C., Blake, D.J. and Reid, K.B.M. (1991). Characterization and organization of the genes encoding the A-, B- and C-chains of human complement subcomponent C1q: The complete derived amino acid sequence of human C1q. *Biochem. J.* **274**: 481–490.

Sim, E., Gill, E.W. and Sim, R.B. (1984). Drugs that induce systemic lupus erythematosus inhibit complement component C4. *Lancet* **2**: 422–424.

Smolen, J.S., Klippel, J.H., Penner, E. et al. (1987). HLA-DR antigens in systemic lupus erythematosus: association with specificity of autoantibody responses to nuclear antigens. *Ann. Rheum. Dis.* **46**: 457–462.

So, A.K., Fielder, A.H., Warner, C.A. et al. (1990). DNA polymorphism of major histocompatibility complex class II and class III genes in systemic lupus erythematosus. *Tissue Antigens* **35**: 144–147.

Speirs, C., Fielder, A.H.L., Chapel, H. et al. (1989). Complement system protein C4 and susceptibility to hydralazine- induced systemic lupus erythematosus. *Lancet.* **1**: 922–924.

Sontheimer, R.D., Maddison, P.J., Reichlin, M. et al. (1982). Serologic and HLA associations in subcutaneous lupus erythematosus, a clinical subset of lupus erythematosus. *Ann. Intern. Med.* **97**: 664–671.

Walport, M.J., Black, C.M. and Batchelor, J.R. (1982). The immunogenetics of SLE. *Clin. Rheum. Dis.* **8**: 3–21.

Waxman, F.J., Hebert, L.A., Comacoff, J.B. et al. (1984). Complement depletion accelerates the clearance of immune complexes from the circulation of primates. *J. Clin. Invest.* **74**: 1329–1340.

Wilson, W.A., Scopelitis, E. and Michalski, J.P. (1984). Association of HLA-DR7 with both antibody to

SS-A (Ro) and disease susceptibility in blacks with systemic lupus erythematosus. *J. Rheumatol.* **11**: 653–657.

Yokohari, R. and Tsunematsu, T. (1985). Application, to Japanese patients, of the 1982 American Rheumatism Association revised criteria for the classification of systemic lupus erythematosus. *Arthritis Rheum.* **28**: 693–698.

Yu, C.Y., Belt, K.T., Giles, C.M. et al. (1986). Structural basis of the polymorphism of human complement components C4A and C4B gene size, reactivity and antigenicity. *EMBO J.* **5**: 2873–2881.

Yu, C.Y. and Campbell, R.D. (1987). Definitive RFLP's to distinguish between the human complement C4A/C4B isotypes and the major Rodgers/Chido determinants: application to the study of C4 null alleles. *Immunogen.* **25**: 383–389.

CHAPTER 9

The contribution of novel MHC genes to disease

John Trowsdale, Stephen Powis
and Duncan Campbell

*Human Immunogenetics Laboratory, Imperial Cancer Research Fund,
London, UK; Department of Biochemistry, MRC Immunochemistry Unit,
Oxford, UK*

Introduction

This volume is mainly concerned with the wealth of information linking immunological disorders with HLA polymorphisms. In this chapter, some of the HLA-linked diseases which do not have an obvious immunological basis are discussed. Some of these, such as 21-hydroxylase deficiency, are clearly explained by known genes within the MHC. In other diseases, such as narcolepsy, the HLA link remains puzzling and may be explained by undiscovered genes, not necessarily involved with the immune system. Some of the novel MHC genes which are thought to be involved in antigen processing will be reviewed and discussed as possible candidates for disease susceptibility loci.

Over 80 genes have now been defined in the 3.6 million bp (3.6 mbp) HLA region (Trowsdale et al., 1991). The most dense area so far, the class III region, contains a gene every 20 kb of DNA, so that the upper limit on the total number of genes in the MHC is $4 \times 10^6/2 \times 10^4$, or 200 genes. The current map of the HLA region is illustrated in Figure 1.1. The class I region has not been explored in as much detail and contains regions of up to 600 kb in which genes have not been identified yet. It is likely that most of the genes in the class II–class III regions have been identified. This degree of definition means it may soon be possible to explain the contribution of the HLA region to most diseases associated with it. The MHC therefore provides an excellent model for analysis of the genetic basis of disease susceptibility, a major focus of biomedical research in this decade.

HLA and Disease
ISBN 0–12–440320–4

Non-immune diseases

There are several diseases strongly associated with the HLA region without an obvious immune aetiology. These include: narcolepsy, idiopathic haemachromatosis and 21-hydroxylase deficiency.

Narcolepsy

Narcolepsy is a sleep disorder of unknown cause. Sufferers are prone to bouts of involuntary sleep, but the clinical definition should include cataplexy as a symptom of true narcolepsy. The disease exhibits the strongest known HLA and disease association. In all populations studied so far, over 98% of affected individuals carry the DRw15-Dw2/DQw1 haplotype (DRB1*1501, DQA1*0102, DQB1*0602). Restriction fragment length polymorphism (RFLP) studies have not identified disease-specific fragments but have confirmed the association with the Dw2 subtype. Interestingly, this is also true for the Japanese population, where the Dw2 subtype represents a minority of DRw15 haplotypes (Juji et al., 1983). Sequences of the DQ and DR genes from narcoleptic individuals reveal no significant differences from normals (Lock et al., 1988; Uryu et al., 1989).

It is not clear whether the primary association is with the class II genes on the DR15-Dw2/DQw1 haplotype or a linked gene, because of the strong linkage between DQ and DR and the lack of any families with recombination in the region. The small number of non-DRw15 cases in the literature do not help to define the causative gene because they possess a variety of DQ and DR types. However, a number of cases of American blacks have now been described which type as DR5 but which have the DQB1*0602 allele in common with the Dw2 haplotype (C. Lock and E. Mignot, personal communication).

Given the current data, there are two alternative hypotheses for the association of narcolepsy with the class II region:

(1) The disease is autoimmune in character and one of the class II products is necessary (but not sufficient) for its development. An autoimmune aetiology has been supported recently by the finding of an association of canine narcolepsy with a µ immunoglobulin switch-like region probe polymorphism (Mignot et al., 1991). The data do not necessarily implicate the switch region itself, rather a gene on a fragment that cross-hybridizes with the probe (E. Mignot and C. Grumet, personal communication). A claim that sleep may be affected in experimental animals by a variety of substances associated with immune responses to bacterial infections, including muramyl peptides, lipopolysaccharide and interleukins adds weight to the notion that the immune system is involved (Krueger and Karnovsky, 1987; Krueger et al., 1990). It has been proposed that these immune-related substances may regulate sleep by altering levels of prostaglandins D2 and E2, with involvement of appropriate neurotransmitters (Hayaishi, 1991). There is also a claim that B cells from DRw15/DQw1 individuals differ in respect to class II-specific binding of muramyl peptides (Silverman et al., 1990).

(2) There may be a non-HLA gene encoding a product affecting sleep, tightly linked to the DR region, which is altered in the DRw15 haplotype. Because of the almost

absolute DRw15 association, such a gene would have to be within, or very close to, the DQw1–DRw15 interval.

Idiopathic haemachromatosis

Hereditary haemachromatosis is an inherited iron storage disease believed to be due to a defect in expression of ferritin in intestinal mucosa (Bothwell et al., 1983). Ferritin is a complex protein which consists of two subunit types, H and L, both of which are derived from multiple gene families scattered on many chromosomes. Only single functional genes have been identified for H and L, on chromosomes 11 and 19, respectively, and there appear to be multiple pseudogenes (Drysdale, 1988; Dugast et al., 1990).

The disease is strongly associated with HLA-A3 in all of the studied Caucasian patients from a variety of countries, and the study populations may be mainly Celtic in origin. The consensus of mapping experiments places the gene within about 1 cM on either side of HLA-A (see Lalouel et al., 1985; Jouanolle et al., 1990, and references therein). Problems in mapping derive partly from difficulties in obtaining precise diagnoses and partly from aberrations in cloning the region telomeric of HLA-A. This observation may be connected with the high rate of recombination in the same region.

Haemochromatosis is widely believed to be due to a non-HLA gene and the finding of ferritin H sequences close to the MHC on the 6p chromosomal segment is of obvious interest (Simon et al., 1987). Two ferritin-related genes have been found on 6p (Dugast et al., 1990). One of them maps to 6p12 and is a non-functional pseudogene. The status and precise position of the other gene is being determined.

21-Hydroxylase deficiency

Two copies of the gene encoding the 21-hydroxylase enzyme, CYP21A and CYP21B, are found in the class III region, lying 3kb downstream of each C4 gene (Carroll et al., 1985; White et al., 1985). The CYP21B gene is active while the CYP21A gene is a highly homologous pseudogene (Higashi et al., 1986; Rodrigues et al., 1987). The presence of the CYP21B gene in the class III region and the demonstration of defects or deletion of the CYP21B gene in patients with congenital adrenal hyperplasia explains the HLA association of this disease (White et al., 1987).

Other diseases

Amongst the large selection of other MHC-linked diseases, there are reports of some cancers. In fact, the first HLA association to be described was with Hodgkin's lymphoma and recent work has localized this to the DP region (Bodmer et al., 1989). It will be of interest to see whether this disease is affected by an immune mechanism. The same could be said for a recent demonstration of a high risk of squamous cell carcinoma of the cervix in women with HLA-DQw3 where there is a strong suggestion of viral involvement and HPV-16 is present in the tumours of up to 90% of affected individuals (Wank and Thomssen, 1991). Recent work has demonstrated a linkage of juvenile myoclonic epilepsy to HLA markers (Greenberg and Delgado-Escueta, 1987; Weissenbecker et al., 1991). A form of autosomal dominant spinocerebellar ataxia is known to be linked to a marker associated with the HLA region, D6S89 (Zoghbi et al., 1989), although probably several cM away, at 6p22.

There was early work suggesting linkage of spina bifida with the MHC, a concept that was stimulated by the linkage of the *t*-complex, with its short-tail phenotype, to the H-2 complex in the mouse. Mapping of some of the orthologous *t* complex genes has been performed in man. The mouse *t* complex consists of two large and two small inversions. So far, the genes studied from the distal inversion are located on human chromosome 6p, in the same order as genes in the *t* haplotype in the mouse (Blanche et al., 1991). Markers on the proximal inversion, such as *TCP-1*, are located on the tip of human chromosome 6q (Willison et al., 1987).

It has been proposed for some time that the driving force for generation of polymorphism was resistance to infectious diseases but it has not been as easy to demonstrate a linkage of the common modern diseases with HLA markers. However, a recent report shows a convincing demonstration of protection against malaria in Africa with particular class I (HLA-B53) and class II (DRB1*1302-DQB1*0501) variants (Hill et al., 1991; Howard, 1991).

Novel MHC genes

The class II region

The human class II region has been completely cloned in yeast artificial chromosomes (YACs) and is partially covered by overlapping cosmids (Ragoussis et al., 1991). Pulse-field gel electrophoresis (PFGE) mapping studies have been used to identify HTF islands (stretches of genomic sequences where there is no suppression of the CpG dinucleotide) between the known class II genes. These islands are generally associated with the 5' ends of genes and novel transcripts have indeed been shown to be derived from some of them (Hanson et al., 1991). Other genes have been located in regions devoid of CpG clusters. In order to identify the genes, probes were made from cosmids and were prehybridized with total human carrier DNA to compete out repeat sequences. These probes were then applied to cDNA libraries to identify expressed sequences. The cDNA probes were then mapped back to the cosmids and characterized by probing on to Northern blots. Several newly described genes have been isolated in this way, the so-called RING series.

The first cluster, centromeric of DP, includes a collagen gene (COL11A2) (Hanson et al., 1989), the human equivalents of previously described mouse genes (KE3 and KE5) (Abe et al., 1988), plus three other genes (RING1, 2 and 5). RING5 is equivalent to a mouse gene centromeric of H-2K, called KE4 (Abe et al., 1988). The RING1 gene contains a conserved motif of cysteine and histidine residues which is also found in a group of proteins including the human immunoglobulin V(D)J recombination activating gene RAG-1. This motif may have some similarities to zinc finger protein sequences and it may define a new family of metal-dependent DNA binding proteins (Hanson et al., 1989; Freemont et al., 1991). So far, none of the genes centromeric of DP are obviously associated functionally with the immune system. Mice have two class I H-2K genes in this position. This arrangement is due to a simple insertion of about 60 kb of DNA containing the K genes, as the two genes flanking H-2K in the mouse, KE3 and RING1, are adjacent in man (Hanson and Trowsdale, 1991).

RING3 is another new gene, at an HTF island 30 kb telomeric of the *HLA-DNA* gene, expressed in a wide variety of tissues. The sequence of this gene is related to that of a *Drosophila* gene, female sterile homeotic, or *fsh*, as well as to some other genes encoding proteins which may be involved in cell division (unpublished data; Haynes et al., 1989). Perhaps mutations in the RING3 gene will exhibit a developmental phenotype in humans. Spies et al. (1990) also located two genes, Y4 and 5 in the position of the RING3 gene. Y4 may be identical to RING3.

Warner et al. (1987b) have reported linkage of a preimplantation-embryo-development (*Ped*) gene to the mouse MHC. They proposed that *Ped* was a Qa-2 product because of a correlation between a *Ped* allele and absence of Qa-2 antigens (Warner et al., 1987a). The other possible developmental phenotype associated with the MHC is multiple recurrent abortion. This seems to be associated with some haplotype combinations, or haplotype sharing which could imply an underlying immune mechanism or simply inbreeding (Tiwari and Terasaki, 1985; Schacter et al., 1979).

Twenty-five kb centromeric of the *DOB* gene, a second HTF island contains genes belonging to the ABC superfamily of transporters (Spies et al., 1990; Trowsdale et al., 1990; Powis et al., 1992). This class of transporters are known to translocate substrates which include peptides and proteins across membranes (Higgins et al., 1990). It has been proposed that the *TAP 1* and *TAP 2* gene products (previously RING4 or PSFI and RING11 or PSF2) form a heterodimer which takes peptides from the cytoplasm across the endoplasmic reticulum (ER) membrane where they meet MHC molecules (see Parham, 1990, and references therein). Evidence that mutations in this region of the MHC affect processing has been provided by studies of mutant cell lines, with defects in peptide presentation through class I molecules, associated with defective expression of these genes (Townsend et al., 1989; Spies and DeMars, 1991; Kelly et al., 1992). In addition, the transporter genes are polymorphic, raising the possibility that some HLA-associated diseases may be linked to the possession of particular alleles of the transporter genes. Similar genes have been found in mice and rats (Monaco et al., 1990; Deverson et al., 1990) and there is a recent claim of a possible association with diabetes, correlating with a reduced level of class I on the cell surface (Faustman et al., 1991). A similar cluster of genes has been identified between *Pb* and *Ob* in the mouse, consistent with conservation of order of the novel genes in the two species (Cho et al., 1991; Hanson and Trowsdale, 1991).

Between the transporter genes is a gene which shares homology with a group of low molecular weight protein constituents of a large protein complex called the proteasome (also known as macropain or multi-catalytic protease, or MCP). Several years ago, work from John Monaco's laboratory revealed two proteasome-like component genes in the MHC class II region, which he called low molecular weight polypeptides (LMPs) (Monaco and McDevitt, 1984, 1986). Given that the proteasome has multiple protease activities it has been proposed that the MHC-encoded members of the complex are involved in producing peptides to feed into the transporter in the

ER (Parham, 1990; Glynne et al., 1991). Two proteasome genes have now been located in mice and humans, now officially called *LMP2* and *LMP7*.

Finding a cluster of genes in the class II region which affect presentation of peptides through class I molecules may influence linkage disequilibrium observed in the region. It also implies that genes within the class II region may play a role in diseases thought to be due simply to the inheritance of particular class I alleles. Since the transporter genes are polymorphic it would not be surprising if different variants affected the presentation of peptides through class I. This kind of scenario could account for the weak class I/class II linkage disequilibrium that is sometimes observed on 'extended haplotypes'. Polymorphism of the *LMP* genes is very limited in humans but there are two variants of each in the mouse (Monaco and McDevitt, 1984, 1986).

Monaco's laboratory also found two new class II-related genes in the class II region (Cho et al., 1991). These are present in man, called *HLA-DMA* and *B* (previously RING6 and RING7) (Kelly et al., 1991). The genes and their products appear to have a class II-related structure, but their sequences are almost as homologous to class I as they are to class II genes.

Thus, there are three types of novel gene emerging in the class II region: (1) genes with no known immune function and no obvious relationship with the MHC (so far, these include RING1 and RING3); (2) genes with a possible immune function, such as peptide generation (*LMP2* and *7*) or transport (*TAP1* and *2*); and (3) new class II genes (*DMA* and *B*) (so far, none of the new genes within the class II region have any known association with disease).

The Class III Region

The class III region is the most extensively cloned region of the MHC and has now been covered by overlapping cosmids (Sargent et al., 1989; Spies et al., 1989a, 1989b; Kendall et al., 1990) and YAC clones (Ragoussis et al., 1991). The organization of this region is illustrated in Figure 1.1. The complement genes are contained in a 120 kb stretch of DNA (Carroll et al., 1984) in the order centromere-*C4B-C4A-Bf-C2*-telomere, with the *C4B* gene lying ~ 400 kb from *DRA*, while the C2 gene lies ~ 600 kb from *HLA-B* (Dunham et al., 1987). This cluster also contains the *CYP21* gene, encoding the 21-hydroxylase enzyme, and the *CYP21P* pseudogene which lie immediately 3' of the *C4B* and *C4A* genes, respectively (Carroll et al., 1985; White et al., 1985; Higashi et al., 1986; Rodrigues et al., 1987). Recently three novel genes have been located in the complement cluster, the *RD*, *G11* and *OSG* genes (Figure 1.1). The *RD* gene (Levi-Strauss et al., 1988) was originally defined in the S region of the mouse H-2 complex by using genomic cosmid fragments in Southern blot analysis to look for evolutionary conservation of sequence between species. The *RD* gene was mapped to a position immediately adjacent to the *Bf* gene in mouse and human cosmids. The *RD* gene spans 6 kb of DNA, and is split into 10 exons which encode a 1.6 kb mRNA. The putative RD protein is a 42 kD intracellular protein with a central core of 52 amino acids consisting of a dipeptide repeat made up of a basic residue (Arg or Lys) next to an acidic one (Asp or Glu). The function of the RD protein is unknown though the mRNA has been detected in all cell lines so far examined, thereby indicating that it may encode a housekeeping protein.

The second novel gene in this region (*OSG*) has been located immediately adjacent to the *CYP21* gene (Morel et al., 1989). In this case the gene is encoded on the opposite strand to that encoding *CYP21* and overlaps with the 3′ end of the *CYP21* gene. The size of the *OSG* has not yet been reported, but it encodes mRNAs of 3.5 kb and 1.8 kb that are expressed in adrenal tissue. A 2.7 kb incomplete cDNA clone appears to specify a protein characterized by the presence of fibronectin type III repeats that show significant homology to tenascin (Matsumoto et al., 1992), a large glycoprotein found in extracellular matrices (Erickson and Bordon, 1989). The *OSG* is part of the unit of duplication at the *C4* loci and part of the sequence is contained between the *CYP21P* and *C4B* genes. Whether this segment of DNA is expressed as mRNA or protein remains to be established.

The third novel gene, *G11*, has been located immediately upstream of the *C4A* gene (Sargent et al., 1989) (Figure 1.1). In this case the gene was identified by establishing the location of an HTF-island ∼10 kb telomeric of the *C4A* gene. Isolation of cDNA clones revealed that the gene spans ∼9.5 kb of DNA and encodes a 1.4 kb mRNA expressed in monocytes, macrophages, T cells, B cells and liver cells. The 3′ end of this gene is part of the unit of duplication of the *C4* genes and ∼0.9 kb of the gene is located immediately upstream of the *C4B* gene (Sargent, 1988; Anderson, 1990). In this case it is not clear whether this segment of sequence is expressed at the mRNA level. The *G11* gene encodes a 28 kD protein, but its function is not known.

In addition to the complement genes which are involved in the humoral immune response, other genes within the class III region that have functions associated with the immune system, include the tumour necrosis factors (*TNF*) *A* and *B* genes (Carroll et al., 1987; Dunham et al., 1987). The *TNF A* and *B* genes are about 1.2 kb apart (Nedospasov et al., 1985) and lie about 220 kb centromeric of the *HLA-B* gene. In addition, three genes encoding members of the heat-shock protein HSP70 family are located between *C2* and the *TNF* genes, 92 kb telomeric of the *C2* gene (Sargent et al., 1989; Milner and Campbell, 1990). Nucleotide sequence analysis of the two intronless genes, *HSP70-1* and *HSP70-2*, which lie 12 kb apart, has shown that they encode an identical protein product of 641 amino acids (Milner and Campbell, 1990). The third intronless gene *HSP70-Hom*, which is located 4 kb telomeric of the *HSP70-1* gene, encodes a more basic protein of 641 amino acids which has 90% sequence similarity with *HSP70-1*. The *HSP70-1* and *HSP70-2* genes are expressed at high levels as an ∼2.4 kb mRNA in cells heat shocked at 42°C. *HSP70-1* is also expressed constitutively at very low levels. The *HSP70-Hom* gene, which has no heat shock consensus sequence in its 5′ flanking sequence, is expressed as an mRNA of approximately 3 kb at low levels both constitutively and following heat shock. Heat-shock protein products of bacteria and other organisms may be involved in the triggering of autoimmunity (Kaufmann, 1991; Moller, 1991). Immune recognition of HSPs from bacteria or other organisms may lead to cross-reactive autoimmune responses to self-HSPs. This has been suggested as one possible mechanism under-lying some autoimmune reactions. A role for heat-shock products may also be invoked in unfolding proteins prior to antigen presentation (Parham, 1990), and in the intracellular transport of peptides. Recently, polymorphism in the promoter region of the *HSP70-1* gene, and in the coding region of the *HSP70-Hom* gene have been established (Milner and Campbell, 1992). However, the functional consequences of this are unclear.

PFGE mapping in the class III region identified a large number of HTF-islands

(Sargent et al., 1989; Kendall et al., 1990). Two are located within the complement gene cluster and define the 5' ends of the *G11* and *RD* genes, while 12 are located between the *C2* and *TNFA* genes. DNA fragments derived from or close to these HTF-islands detected transcripts in Northern blot analysis, and these together with cosmid genomic inserts have been used as hybridization probes to isolate the corresponding cDNA clones (Sargent et al., 1989; Spies et al., 1989a and 1989b; Kendall et al., 1990). The region between the *C4* and *HLA-DRA* genes has also been shown to contain HTF-islands, where seven have been mapped within a 160 kb stretch of DNA (Kendall et al., 1990). Seven novel genes were identified by the isolation of cDNA clones using cosmid genomic inserts as hybridization probes, and Northern blot analysis, at least five of which appear to be associated with HTF-islands.

So far 36 genes have now been located in a 680 kb stretch of DNA within the class III region (Kendall et al., 1990). A large number of these, 19, are associated with HTF-islands, and appear to be ubiquitously expressed. Intermingled with these genes are genes with tissue-specific expression. The *CYP21B* and *OSG* genes are expressed in the adrenal gland (White et al., 1987; Morel et al., 1989), for example. In addition, one of the novel genes, *G1*, defined by Sargent et al. (1989) appears to have a very restricted expression, the *G1* mRNA being observed only in the monocytoid cell line U937 and the immature leukaemic T-cell line Molt4. Thus the cloned region and the remaining segment yet to be cloned may contain several more genes which are expressed in a tissue specific manner.

Sequence analysis of cDNA clones corresponding to some of the novel genes have now begun to reveal what they encode. For example, the single copy *G7a* gene encodes a 1265 amino-acid protein of molecular weight 140 kD (Hsieh and Campbell, 1991). Comparison of the derived amino-acid sequence of *G7a* with protein databases revealed similarity to valyl-tRNA synthetases. The molecular weight of the *G7a* protein is similar to that of other mammalian valyl-tRNA synthetases suggesting that the *G7a* gene codes for the human form of this enzyme. The *G1* gene appears to encode a 93 amino-acid polypeptide which shares 35% identity with the intracellular Ca^{2+}-binding protein calmodulin (Olaveson et al., 1992). This similarity is based around two putative Ca^{2+}-binding sites in the G1 protein and suggests that G1 is a novel Ca^{2+}-binding protein. The *G13* gene has also been characterized and appears to encode a 77 kD protein (Khanna and Campbell, 1992) that shows homology with the cyclic AMP response element binding protein (CREB) suggesting that *G13* could be a novel type of transcription factor. Two of the other newly described genes in the class III region, *BAT2(G2)* and *BAT3(G3)*, encode large proline-rich proteins of molecular weights 228 kD and 110 kD, respectively (Banerji et al., 1990). These do not appear to be members of any known family of proteins.

Although the functions of *BAT2* and *BAT3* and the proteins encoded by most of the other novel genes mapped in the class III region are yet unknown, some may be involved in different aspects of the immune response. For example, a genetic locus controlling the expression of an alloantigen recognized by natural killer (NK) cells has been mapped between *TNFA* and *H-2S* in the mouse complex (Rembecki et al., 1988a, 1988b). The murine genes may have a human counterpart which has been labelled the *EC1* locus (Ciccione et al., 1990). This locus, which has been mapped between *Factor B* and *HLA-B* loci, governs the susceptibility or resistance to lysis by alloreactive natural killer cells.

Teuscher et al. (1990) have mapped a locus controlling the immune response (Ir) to autoimmune orchitis, designated *Orch-1*, within the *C4/H-2D* segment, by analysing intra-H-2 recombinant congenic mouse strains, while a gene governing the response to TNP-Ficoll has been mapped to the same segment (Hillstrom Shapiro et al., 1985). The mechanism(s) underlying these Ir gene effects are unknown, none the less in view of the strong homology and the phylogenetic conservation of the MHCs of mouse and man, it is possible that in man this region may encode the equivalent genes which are involved in immune function. In addition, data presented by Schaffer et al. (1989), French and Dawkins (1990) and others, suggest that genetic susceptibility to IgA deficiency and common variable immunodeficiency (CVID) appears to be influenced by a gene(s) within the class II region. More recently, by analysing polymorphic markers for 11 genes or their products extending from *HLA-DQ* to *HLA-A*, further support for the hypothesis that a susceptibility gene for both IgA deficiency and CVID is located in the class III region of the MHC has been provided. These genes may be located between the *C4B* and *C2* genes.

The Class I Region

Although the largest area of the MHC, the class I region contains the fewest markers, little is known about any resident non-class I genes. The mouse class I region has been given more attention, but this has exclusively involved studies of the class I genes themselves. These have a variety of expression patterns and may have evolved specialized functions. For example, the M region genes in the mouse appear to encode products which present f-met peptides from mitochondrial proteins or from bacteria (Fischer Lindahl et al., 1990).

Gene clusters

The MHC will provide a useful model for future study of the organization of the human genome. There are several issues which should be resolved in the next few years. For example, it will be of interest to determine if the genes are arranged randomly, or if there is a particular placement of tissue-specific genes, housekeeping genes, HTF islands, repeat sequences, replication points and AT-GC-rich stretches (Ikemura et al., 1992), since little is known about the structure and arrangement of chromatin. Of particular interest as far as the MHC is concerned are the reasons behind clustering of genes with interrelated functions. The two most obvious explanations are co-regulation or co-evolution. This kind of information is of concern for disease studies and may help to explain the high degree of linkage disequilibrium observed in the region.

MHC-linked diseases may have accounted for the marked polymorphism in the region, yet there is little information on which diseases have provided the driving force. Some very interesting observations have been made concerning the mating preference of mice and H-2 type, which provide a mechanism for driving variation into the population. Using the association of MHC alleles with urinary odours, male mice have a tendency to prefer mating with female mice of a different MHC type (Yamazaki et al., 1976). These observations imply that the MHC is the genomic locus whose heterozygosity is of prime concern for fitness of the individual and hence resistance to disease (Howard, 1991; Potts et al., 1991).

References

Abe, K., Wei, J.F., Wei, F.S. et al. (1988). Searching for coding sequences in the mammalian genome: the H-2K region of the mouse MHC is replete with genes expressed in embryos. *EMBO J.* **7**: 3441–3449.

Anderson, M.J. (1990). Molecular genetics of the human complement protein C4. D. Phil. thesis, University of Oxford.

Banerji, J., Sands, J., Strominger, J.L. et al. (1990). A gene pair from the human major histocompatibility complex encodes large proline-rich proteins with multiple repeated motifs and a single ubiquitin-like domain. *Proc. Natl Acad. Sci. USA* **87**: 2374–2378.

Blanche, H., Zoghbi, H.Y., Jabs, E.W. et al. (1991). A centromere-based genetic map of the short arm of human chromosome 6. *Genomics* **9**: 420–428.

Bodmer, J.G., Tonks, S., Oza, A.M. et al. (1989). HLA-DP based resistance to Hodgkin's disease. *Lancet* **2**: 1455–1456.

Bothwell, T.H., Charlton, R.W., Motulsky, A.G. et al. (1983). *The Metabolic Basis of Inherited Disease*, pp. 1269–1298, McGraw-Hill, New York.

Carroll, M.C., Campbell, R.D., Bentley, D.R. et al. (1984). A molecular map of the human major histocompatibility complex class III region linking complement genes C4, C2 and Factor B. *Nature* **307**: 237–241.

Carroll, M.C., Campbell, R.D. and Porter, R.R. (1985). Mapping of steroid 21-hydroxylase genes adjacent to complement component C4 genes in HLA, the major histocompatibility complex in man. *Proc. Natl Acad. Sci. USA* **82**: 521–525.

Carroll, M.C., Katzman, P., Alicot, E.M. et al. (1987). Linkage map of the human major histocompatibility complex including the tumor necrosis factor genes. *Proc. Natl Acad. Sci. USA* **84**: 8535–8539.

Cho, S., Attaya, M., Brown, M.G. et al. (1991). A cluster of transcribed sequences between the Pb and Ob genes of the murine major histocompatibility complex. *Proc. Natl Acad. Sci. USA* **88**: 5197–5201.

Cho, S., Attaya, M. and Monaco, J.J. (1991). New class II-like genes in the murine MHC. *Nature* **353**: 573–576.

Ciccione, E., Colonna, M., Viale, O. et al. (1990). Susceptibility or resistance to lysis by alloreactive natural killer cells is governed by a gene in the human major histocompatibility complex between Bf and HLA-B. *Proc. Natl Acad. Sci. USA* **87**: 9794–9797.

Deverson, E.V., Gow, I.R., Coadwell, J. et al. (1990). MHC class II region encoding proteins related to the multidrug resistance family of transmembrane transporters. *Nature* **348**: 738–741.

Drysdale, J.W. (1988). Human ferritin gene expression. *Prog. Nucleic Acid Res. Mol. Biol.* **35**: 5127–5155.

Dugast, I.J., Papadopoulos, P., Zaffone, E. et al. (1990). Identification of two human ferritin H genes on the short arm of chromosome 6. *Genomics* **6**: 204–211.

Dunham, I., Sargent, C.A., Trowsdale, J. et al. (1987). Molecular mapping of the human major histocompatibility complex by pulsed-field gel electrophoresis. *Proc. Natl Acad. Sci. USA* **84**: 7237–7241.

Erickson, H.P. and Bordon, M.A. (1989). Tenascin an extracellular matrix protein prominent in specialized embryonic tissues and turnouts. *Annu. Rev. Cell. Biol.* **5**: 71–92.

Faustman, D., Li, X., Herbert, Y. et al. (1991). Linkage of faulty major histocompatibility complex class I to autoimmune diabetes. *Science* **254**: 1756–1761.

Fischer Lindahl, K., Hermal, E., Loveland, B.E. et al. (1990). Molecular definition of a mitochondrially encoded mouse minor histocompatibility antigen. *Cold Spring Harb. Symp. Quant. Biol.* **54**: 563–568.

Freemont, P.S., Hanson, I.M., Trowsdale, J. et al. (1991). A novel cysteine-rich sequence motif. *Cell* **64**: 483–484.

French, M.A.H. and Dawkins, R.L. (1990). Central MHC genes, IgA deficiency and autoimmune disease. *Immunol. Today* **11**: 271–274.

Glynne, R., Powis, S.H., Beck, S. et al. (1991). A proteasome-related gene between the two ABC transporter loci in the class II region of the human MHC. *Nature* **353**: 357–360.

Greenberg, D.A. and Delgado-Escueta, A.V. (1987). A locus involved in the expression of juvenile myoclonic epilepsy and of an associated EEG trait may be linked to HLA and Bf. *Cytogenet. Cell Genet.* **46**: 623–628.

Hanson, I.M., Gorman, P., Lui, V.C.H. et al. (1989). The human alpha 2(XI) collagen gene (COL11A2) maps to the centromeric border of the major histocompatibility complex on chromosome 6. *Genomics* **5**: 925–931.

Hanson, I.M., Poustka, A., Trowsdale, J. et al. (1991). New genes in the class II region of the human major histocompatibility complex. *Genomics* **10**: 417–424.

Hanson, I.M. and Trowsdale, J. (1991). Colinearity of novel genes in the class II regions of the MHC in mouse and human. *Immunogenet.* **34**: 5–11.

Hayaishi, O. (1991). Molecular mechanisms of sleep-wake regulation: roles of prostaglandins D2 and E2. *FASEB* **5**: 2575–2581.

Haynes, S.R., Mozer, B.A., Bhatia-Day, N. et al. (1989). The Drosophila fsh locus, a maternal effect homeotic gene, encodes apparent membrane proteins. *Dev. Biol.* **134**: 246–257.

Higashi, Y., Yoshioka, H., Yamane, M. et al. (1986). Complete nucleotide sequence of two steroid 21-hydroxylase genes tandemly arranged in human chromosome: a pseudogene and a genuine gene. *Proc. Natl Acad. Sci. USA* **83**: 2841–2845.

Higgins, C.F., Hyde, S.C., Mimmack, M.M. et al. (1990). Binding protein-dependent transport systems. *J. Bioerg. Biomem.* **22**: 571–592.

Hill, A.V.S., Allsop, C.E.M., Kwiatkowski, D. et al. (1991). Common West African HLA antigens are associated with protection from severe malaria. *Nature* **352**: 595–600.

Hillstrom Shapiro, L., Dugan, E.S. and Neiderhuber, J.E. (1985). Monoclonal antibody characterization of a unique immune response control locus between H-2S and D. *J. Exp. Med.* **162**: 1477–1493.

Howard, J.C. (1991). Disease and evolution. *Nature* **352**: 565–567.

Hsieh, S.L. and Campbell, R.D. (1991). Evidence that gene G7a in the human major histocompatibility complex is valyl-tRNA synthetase. *Biochem. J.* **278**: 809–816.

Ikemura, T., Matsumoto, K., Ishihara, N. et al. (1992). Giant G+C% mosaic structures in the HLA locus and a border between the mosaic domains. In *HLA 1991* (eds K. Tsuji, M. Aizawa and T. Sasazuki), Oxford University Press, Oxford.

Jouanolle, A.M., Yaouanq, J., Blayan, M. et al. (1990). HLA class I gene polymorphism in genetic hemochromatosis. *Hum. Genet.* **85**: 279–282.

Juji, T., Satake, M., Honda, Y. et al. (1983). HLA antigens in Japanese patients with narcolepsy: all patients were DR2 positive. *Tissue Antigens* **24**: 316–319.

Kaufmann, S.H.E. (1991). Heat shock proteins and the immune response. In *Current Topics in Microbiology & Immunology*. Springer-Verlag, New York.

Kelly, A.P., Monaco, J.J., Cho, S. et al. (1991). A new human HLA class II-related locus, DM. *Nature* **353**: 571–573.

Kelly, A., Powis, S.H., Kerr, L.-A. et al. (1992). Assembly and function of the two ABC transporter proteins encoded in the human major histocompatibility complex. *Nature* **355**: 641–644.

Kendall, E., Sargent, C.A. and Campbell, R.D. (1990). Human major histocompatibility complex contains a new cluster of genes between the HLA-D and complement C4 loci. *Nucleic Acids Res.* **18**: 7251–7257.

Khanna, A. and Campbell, R.D. (1992). Characterisation of a novel gene G13 in the class III region of the human MHC. In *HLA 1991* (eds K. Tsuji, M. Aizawa and T. Sasazuki), pp. 198–202, Oxford University Press, Oxford.

Krueger, J.M. and Karnovsky, M.L. (1987). Sleep and the immune response. *Ann. N.Y. Acad. Sci.* **496**: 510–516.

Krueger, J.M., Obal, F., Opp, M. et al. (1990). Putative sleep neuromodulators. In *Sleep and Biological Rhythms.* pp. 163–185, Oxford University Press, Oxford.

Lalouel, J.M., Le Mignon, L., Simon, M. et al. (1985). Genetic analysis of idiopathic hemochromatosis using both qualitative (disease status) and quantitative (serm iron) information. *Am. J. Hum. Genet.* **37**: 700–718.

Levi-Strauss, M., Carroll, M.C., Steinmetz, M. et al. (1988). A previously undetected MHC gene with an unusual periodic structure. *Science* **240**: 242–251.

Lock, C.B., So, A.K., Welsh, K.I. et al. (1988). MHC class II sequences of an HLA-DR2 narcoleptic. *Immunogenet.* **27**: 449–455.

Matsumoto, K., Arai, M., Ishi Hara, N. et al. (1992). Cluster of fibronectin type-III repeats found in the human major histocompatibility complex class III region shows the highest homology with the repeats in an extracellular matrix protein, tenascin. *Genomics* **12**: 485–491.

Mignot, E., Wang, C., Rattazzi, C. et al. (1991). Genetic linkage of autosomal recessive canine narcolepsy with a μ immunoglobulin heavy-chain switch-like segment. *Proc. Natl Acad. Sci. USA* **88**: 3475–3478

Milner, C.M. and Campbell, R.D. (1990). Structure and expression of the three MHC-linked HSP70 genes. *Immunogenetics* **32**: 242–251.

Milner, C.M. and Campbell, R.D. (1992). Polymorphic analysis of the three MHC-linked HSP70 genes in *HLA 1991* (eds K. Tsuji, M. Aizawa and T. Sasazuki), pp. 157–161, Oxford University Press, Oxford.

Moller, G. (1991). *Heat Shock Proteins and the Immune System*. Immunological Reviews 22, Munksgaard, Copenhagen.

Monaco, J.J. and McDevitt, H.O. (1984). H-2 linked low-molecular weight polypeptide antigens assemble into an unusual macromolecular complex. *Nature* **309**: 797–799.

Monaco, J.J. and McDevitt, H.O. (1986). The LMP antigens: a stable MHC-controlled multisubunit protein complex. *Hum. Immunol.* **15**: 416–426.

Monaco, J.J., Cho, S., Attaya, M. et al. (1990). Transport protein genes in the murine MHC. *Science* **250**: 1723–1726.

Morel, Y., Bristow, J., Gitelman, S.E. et al. (1989). Transcript encoded on the opposite strand of the human steroid 21-hydroxylase/complement component C4 gene locus. *Proc. Natl Acad. Sci. USA* **86**: 6582–6586.

Nedospasov, S.A., Shakov, A.N., Tivelskaya, R.L. et al. (1985). Molecular cloning of human gene coding tumour necrosis factors: tandem arrangement of α- and β-genes in a short segment (6000 bp) of human genome. *Dokl. Acad. Nauk. SSSR* **285**: 1487–1490.

Olaveson, M.G., Thomson, W., Cheng, J. et al. (1992). Characterisation of a novel gene G1 in the human MHC class III region. In *HLA 1991* (eds K. Tsuji, M. Aizawa and T. Sasazuki), pp. 190–192. Oxford University Press, Oxford.

Parham, P. (1990). Antigen processing. Transporters of delight. *Nature* **348**: 674–675.

Potts, W.K., Manning, C.J. and Wakeland, E.K. (1991). Mating patterns in seminatural populations of mice influenced by MHC genotype. *Nature* **352**: 619–621.

Powis, S.H., Mockridge, I., Kelly, A. et al. (1992). Polymorphism in a second ABC transporter gene located within the class II region of the human MHC. *Proc. Natl Acad. Sci. USA* **89**: 1463–1467.

Ragoussis, J., Monaco, A., Mockridge, I. et al. (1991). Cloning of the HLA class II region in yeast artificial chromosomes. *Proc. Natl Acad. Sci. USA* **88**: 3753–3757.

Rembecki, R.M., Kumar, V., David, C.S. et al. (1988a). Bone marrow cell transplants involving intra-H-2 recombinant inbred mouse strains. Evidence that hemopoietic histocompatibility-1 (Hh-1) genes are distinct from H-2D or H-2L. *J. Immunol.* **141**: 2253–2260.

Rembecki, R.M., Kumar, V., David, C.S. et al. (1988b). Polymorphism of Hh-1, the mouse hemopoietic locus. *Immunogenet.* **28**: 158–170.

Rodriques, N.R., Dunham, I., Yu, C.Y. et al. (1987). Molecular characterization of the HLA-linked steroid 21-hydroxylase B gene from an individual with congenital adrenal hyperplasia. *EMBO J.* **6**: 1653–1661.

Sargent, C.A. (1988). Molecular mapping of the HLA class III region. D. Phil. thesis. University of Oxford.

Sargent, C.A., Dunham, I. and Campbell, R.D. (1989). Identification of multiple HTF-island associated genes in the human major histocompatibility complex class III region. *EMBO J.* **8**: 2305–2312.

Schacter, B., Gyves, M., Muir, A. et al. (1979). HLA-A,B compatibility in parents of offspring with neural-tube defects or couples experiencing involuntary fetal wastage. *Lancet* **1**: 796–799.

Schaffer, F.M., Palermos, J., Zhu, Z-B. et al. (1989). Individuals with IgA deficiency and common variable immunodeficiency share polymorphisms of major histocompatibility complex class III genes. *Proc. Natl Acad. Sci. USA* **86**: 8015–8019.

Silverman, D.H., Sayegh, M.H., Alvarez, C.E. et al. (1990). HLA class II-restricted binding of muramyl peptides to B lymphocytes of normal and narcoleptic subjects. *Hum. Immunol.* **27**: 145–154.

Simon, M., LeMignon, L., Fauchet, R. et al. (1987). A study of 609 HLA haplotypes marking for the hemochromatosis gene: (1) Mapping of the gene near the HLA-A locus and characters required to define a heterozygous population and (2) hypothesis concerning the underlying cause of hemochromatosis-HLA association. *Am. J. Hum. Genet.* **41**: 89–105.

Spies, T. and DeMars, R. (1991). Restored expression of major histocompatibility class I molecules by gene transfer of a putative peptide transporter. *Nature* **351**: 323–324.

Spies, T., Blanck, G., Bresnahan, M. et al. (1989a). A new cluster of genes within the human major histocompatibility complex. *Science* **243**: 214–217.

Spies, T., Bresnahan, M., Strominger, J.L. et al. (1989b). Human major histocompatibility complex contains a minimum of 19 genes between the complement cluster and HLA-B. *Proc. Natl Acad. Sci. USA* **86**: 8955–8598.

Spies, T., Bresnahan, M., Bahram, S. et al. (1990). A gene in the human major histocompatibility complex class II region controlling the class I antigen presentation pathway. *Nature* **348**: 744–747.

Teuscher, C., Gasser, D.L., Woodland, S.R. et al. (1990). Experimental allergic orchitis in mice. VI. Recombinations within the H-2S/H-2D interval define the maop position of the H-2-associated locus controlling disease susceptibility. *Immunogenet.* **32**: 337–344.

Tiwari, J.L. and Terasaki, P.I. (1985). *HLA and Disease*. Springer-Verlag, New York.

Townsend, A., Ohlen, C., Foster, L. et al. (1989). A mutant cell in which association of class I heavy and light chains is induced by viral peptides. *Cold Spring Harb. Symp. Quant. Biol.* LIV: 299–308.

Trowsdale, J., Hanson, I., Mockridge, I. et al. (1990). Sequences encoded in the class II region of the MHC related to the ABC superfamily of transporters. *Nature* **348**: 741–744.

Trowsdale, J., Ragoussis, J. and Campbell, R.D. (1991). Map of the human MHC. *Immunol. Today* **12**: 443–446.

Uryu, N., Maeda, M., Nagata, Y. et al. (1989). No difference in the nucleotide sequence of the DQbeta beta 1 domain between narcoleptic and healthy individuals with DR2, Dw2. *Hum. Immunol.* **24**: 175–181.

Wank, R. and Thomssen, M. (1991). High risk of squamous cell carcinoma of the cervix for women with HLA-DQw3. *Nature* **352**: 723–725.

Warner, C.M., Gollnick, S.O., Flaherty, L. et al. (1987a). Analysis of Qa-2 antigen expression by preimplantation mouse embryos: possible relationship to the proimplantation-embryo-development (Ped) gene product. *Biol. Reprod.* **36**: 611–616.

Warner, C.M., Gollnick, S.O., Goldbarb, S.B. et al. (1987b). Linkage of the proimplantation-embryo-development (Ped) gene to the mouse major histocompatibility complex (MHC). *Biol. Reprod.* **36**: 606–610.

Weissenbecker, K.A., Durner, M., Scaramelli, A. et al. (1991). Confirmation of linkage between juvenile myoclonic epilepsy and the HLA region of chromosome 6. *Am. J. Med. Genet.* **38**: 32–36.

White, P.C., New, M.I. and Dupont, B. (1987). Congenital adrenal hyperplasia. *N. Engl. J. Med.* **316**: 1519–1524.

White, P.C., Grossberger, D., Onufer, B.J. et al. (1985). Two genes encoding steroid 21-hydroxylase are located near the genes encoding the fourth component of complement in man. *Proc. Natl Acad. Sci. USA* **82**: 1089–1093.

Willison, K., Kelly, A., Dudley, K. et al. (1987). The human homologue of the mouse t-complex gene, TCP1, is located on chromosome 6 but is not near the HLA region. *EMBO J.* **6**: 1967–1974.

Yamazaki, K., Boyse, E.A., Mike, V. et al. (1976). Control of mating preferences in mice by genes in the major histocompatibility complex. *J. Exp. Med.* **144**: 1324–1335.

Zoghbi, H., Sandkuyl, L., Ott, J. et al. (1989). Assignment of autosomal dominant spinocerebellar ataxia (SCA1) centromeric to the HLA region on the short arm of chromosome 6, using multilocus analysis. *Am. J. Hum. Genet.* **44**: 255–263.

Index